Applied Radiological Anatomy for Medical Students

Applied Radiological Anatomy for Medical Students is the definitive atlas of human anatomy, utilizing the complete range of imaging modalities to describe normal anatomy and radiological findings.

Initial chapters describe all imaging techniques and introduce the principles of image interpretation. These are followed by comprehensive sections on each antomical region.

Hundreds of high-quality radiographs, MRI, CT and ultrasound images are included, complemented by concise, focused text. Many images are accompanied by detailed, fully labeled, line illustrations to aid interpretation.

Written by leading experts and experienced teachers in imaging and anatomy, *Applied Radiological Anatomy for Medical Students* is an invaluable resource for all students of anatomy and radiology.

PAUL BUTLER is a Consultant Neuroradiologist at The Royal London Hospital, London.

ADAM W. M. MITCHELL is a Consultant Radiologist at Charing Cross Hospital, London.

HAROLD ELLIS is a Clinical Anatomist at the University of London.

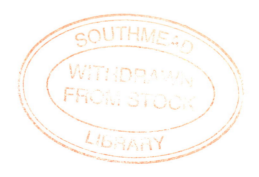

Applied Radiological

Anatomy for Medical Students

Edited by

PAUL BUTLER
The Royal London Hospital

ADAM W. M. MITCHELL
Charing Cross Hospital

HAROLD ELLIS
University of London

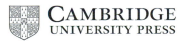
CAMBRIDGE
UNIVERSITY PRESS

CAMBRIDGE UNIVERSITY PRESS
Cambridge, New York, Melbourne, Madrid, Cape Town, Singapore, São Paulo, Delhi

Cambridge University Press
The Edinburgh Building, Cambridge CB2 8RU, UK

Published in the United States of America by Cambridge University Press, New York

www.cambridge.org
Information on this title: www.cambridge.org/9780521819398

First published 2007
Reprinted 2009

Printed in the United Kingdom at the University Press, Cambridge

A catalog record for this publication is available from the British Library

ISBN 978-0-521-81939-8 paperback

Contents

Contributors

ALEX M. BARNACLE
Department of Radiology, Charing Cross Hospital, London, UK

JONATHAN D. BERRY
Department of Radiology, King's College Hospital, London, UK

JOTI BHATTACHARYA MRCP FRCR
Institute of Neurological Sciences, Southern General Hospital, Glasgow, UK

DOMINIC BLUNT MRCP FRCR
Department of Radiology, Charing Cross Hospital, London, UK

THOMAS H. BRYANT MBCHB MMEDSCI FRCR
Department of Imaging, Hammersmith Hospitals NHS Trust, London, UK

PAUL BUTLER MRCP FRCR
The Royal London Hospital, Department of Neuroradiology, London, UK

STELLA COMITIS MBBCH FRCR
Department of Radiology, Charing Cross Hospital, London, UK

SUJAL R. DESAI MD MRCP FRCR
Department of Radiology, King's College Hospital, London, UK

CLAUDIA KIRSCH BA MD FRCR
Diagnostic Neuroradiology and Head and Neck Radiology, David Geffen School of Medicine at UCLA, Los Angeles CA, USA

ADAM W. M. MITCHELL MBBS FRCS FRCR
Department of Radiology, Charing Cross Hospital, London, UK

A. NEWMAN SANDERS MBBS MRCP FRCR
Department of Diagnostic Imaging, Mayday University Hospital NHS Trust, Thornton Heath, Surrey, UK

IAN SUCHET
Department of Radiology, Charing Cross Hospital, London, UK

ANDREA G. ROCKALL BSC MBBS MRCP FRCR
Department of Radiology, Barts and the London NHS Trust, Barts and The London School of Medicine, Department of Nuclear Medicine, London, UK

JUREERAT THAMMAROJ MD MSC
Srinagarind Hospital, Khon Kaen University, Thailand

SARAH J. VINNICOMBE BSC (HONS) MRCP FRCR
Department of Radiology, Barts and the London NHS Trust, Barts and The London School of Medicine, Department of Nuclear Medicine, London, UK

RUTH WILLIAMSON
Department of Radiology, Charing Cross Hospital, London, UK

ADAM D. WALDMAN PHD MRCP FRCR
Department of Radiology, Charing Cross Hospital, London, UK

Acknowledgments

The editors and publisher wish to acknowledge with thanks the excellent work of Mr. Jack Barber, Dr. Jo Bhattacharya and Dr. Ivan Moseley in the preparation of the line drawings, which illustrate the radiology images. Some of these line drawings have been redrawn and adapted from originals which appeared in *Grant's Atlas of Anatomy* © Williams & Wilkins and from *Langman's Medical Embryology* © Williams & Wilkins and we are grateful for the permission of the publisher to allow their adaptation in this work.

Section 1 | The basics

Chapter 1 | An introduction to the technology of imaging

THOMAS H. BRYANT
and ADAM D. WALDMAN

Introduction

Imaging techniques available to the radiologist are changing rapidly, due largely to advances in imaging and computer technology. Three of the five imaging modalities described in this chapter did not exist in recognizable form 30 years ago. This chapter is a brief overview of the major medical imaging techniques in current use with reference to the underlying principles, equipment, the type of information that they yield, and their advantages and limitations.

X-rays

X-rays were discovered by a physicist named Wilhelm Roentgen in November 1895, using a type of cathode ray tube invented in 1877 by Crooke. With this "new kind of ray," he produced a photograph of his wife's hand showing the bones and her wedding ring, requiring an exposure time of about 30 minutes. Within a month of this discovery, X-rays were being deliberately generated in a number of countries, and were being used for imaging patients by early 1896. A modern X-ray machine is shown in Fig. 1.1.

X-ray generation

The basics of the X-ray tube have remained unchanged since Roentgen's time, although the details have changed. X-rays are made up of photons and are a type of electromagnetic radiation like light or radio-waves, although they have higher energy.

The basic X-ray tube is a vacuum tube (Fig. 1.2). A high voltage is passed through a wire, heating it and allowing electrons to be freed and leave the wire at its surface (the cathode). The electrons are accelerated towards a second electrode with a positive charge (the anode) causing a current to flow between the cathode and anode. If the anode

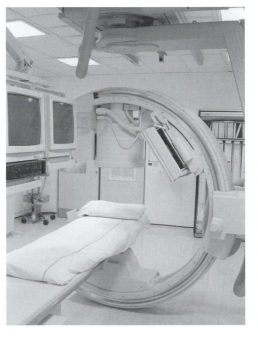

Fig. 1.1. **An example of a fluoroscopy machine that uses X-radiation to produce images of patients. The tube can be rotated around the patient to provide views from different projections. Moving images can be viewed using the image intensifier or static images can be obtained.**

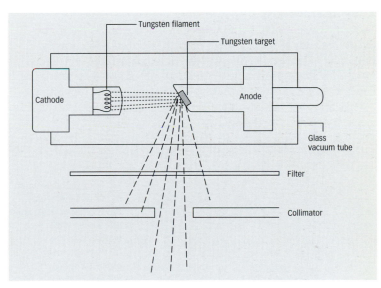

Fig. 1.2. **The essentials of a simple, fixed anode X-ray generation set.**

Applied Radiological Anatomy for Medical Students. Paul Butler, Adam Mitchell, and Harold Ellis (eds.) Published by Cambridge University Press. © P. Butler, A. Mitchell, and H. Ellis 2007.

(a)

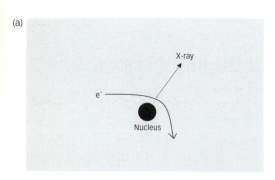

Fig. 1.3. **Diagrams of the production of X-rays.** (a) **Bremsstrahlung or Braking radiation** occurs when the free electron is deflected by the electric field around the nucleus of a target atom, shedding energy in the form of a photon as the free electron is slowed.

(b)

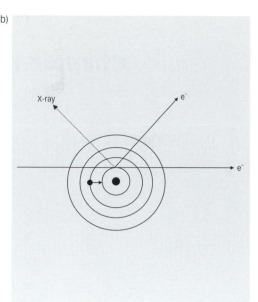

Fig. 1.3. (b) **Characteristic radiation**. When a free electron knocks one of the "cloud" of orbital shell electrons out of an atoms, an electron from a higher energy (outer) shell moves to fill the gap, shedding the excess energy in the form of an electromagnetic photon which will be an X-ray photon if the energies are high enough. These X-rays have an energy specific to the transition between the shells, and the pattern of production is therefore characteristic of the anode material.

is made of the correct material and the electrons are accelerated enough (by at least 1000 volts), X-rays will be produced. Typical materials used for the anode include tungsten and molybdenum, which have high atomic numbers, and high melting points (the X-ray tube gets very hot). Over 90% of the energy supplied is lost as heat.

X-ray photons are produced at the anode when a free electron travelling at high speed interacts with a target atom. Two main interactions occur in the diagnostic X-ray energy range, Bremsstrahlung and characteristic radiation (Fig. 1.3).

The X-rays then leave the tube through a filter (usually made of copper or molybdenum), which removes X-ray photons with undesirable energies, leaving those in the diagnostic range.

Finally, the X-rays pass through a collimator. X-rays produced at the anode travel in all directions, although some features of the design cause them to mainly be directed towards the patient. The collimator is an aperture (usually made of lead) that can be opened and closed so that only the part of the patient to be imaged is exposed to the X-ray beam.

How X-rays produce an image
Production of a radiograph, an X-ray image, is the result of the interaction of X-ray photons with the patient and detection of the remaining photons.

X-ray interactions
There are two main types of interaction that are important in the diagnostic X-ray range (Fig. 1.4). Photoelectric absorption is more important at low energy (low kV) X-ray photon energies and is seen more with elements with high atomic numbers – such as calcium in bones. Compton (incoherent) scattering becomes more important for biological tissues as X-ray photon energies increase (high kV) and is proportional to tissue density.

Detection of X-rays
Following irradiation of the patient, some of the X-rays are absorbed, some are scattered (deflected) and some pass through the patient. These effects depend on the nature and thickness of the tissues in their path.

X-ray photons are invisible. There are a number of mechanisms to detect X-ray photons and convert them to a visible image (Fig. 1.5).

Film
Although photographic film is sensitive to X-rays by itself, fluorescent screens are used inside X-ray cassettes that convert X-ray photons to visible light, decreasing the number of X-ray photons required to make an image and therefore the radiation dose to the patient. The light produced then exposes the photographic film by converting crystals of silver halide into elemental silver. These initial specks of silver are grown during processing, and appear black on the film.

(a)

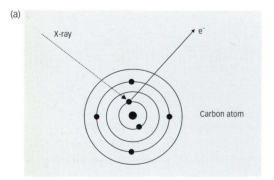

Fig. 1.4. **A representation of the two important types of X-ray (and γ-ray) interaction with biological tissue.** (a) **Photoelectric absorption** occurs when an X-ray photon with sufficient energy is absorbed, breaking the bond of an atomic electron and knocking it out of the electron shell.

(b)

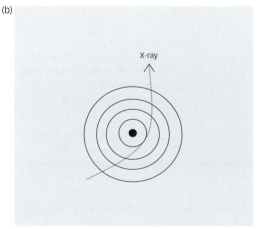

Fig. 1.4. (b) **Compton (incoherent) scattering** occurs when the X-ray photon interacts with an atomic electron, resulting in deflection of the photon with a transfer of kinetic energy to the electron. This is known as scattering as the X-ray photon continues in a different direction (which can even be the reverse of the original direction, in the case of a head on collision).

(a)

(b)

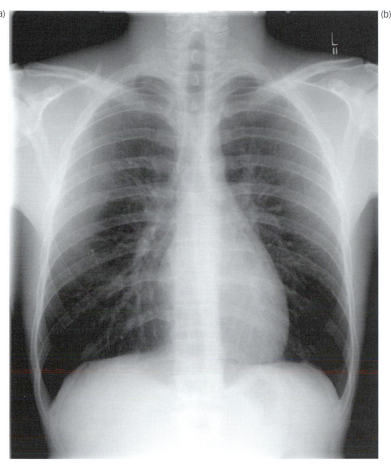
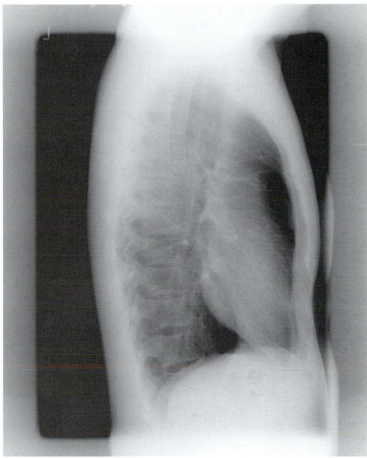

Fig. 1.5. **A radiograph ("plain film") of the chest. This has been acquired on a CR system using an X-ray generation set and europium-activated barium fluorohalide plate read by a laser. Both PA (postero-anterior) and lateral views are shown. The views are named from the direction the X-rays pass through the patient and the location of the detector: in the case of the PA film the X-ray tube is behind the patient and the detector plate in front so the X-rays pass from posterior to anterior.**

Computed radiology (CR)

Special plates are made from europium-activated barium fluoro-halides. These plates absorb the X-ray photons emerging from the patient, storing them as a latent image. The plates are then scanned with a laser, causing emission of light that can be read by a light detecting photo-multiplier tube connected to a computer on which the image can be viewed.

Digital radiology (DR)

A number of devices for direct digital acquisition of images exist. CCD (charged coupled device) technology such as is found in modern digital cameras can be adapted to detect X-rays by coating the device with a visible light producing substance such as cesium iodide or by using a fluorescent screen. TFT (thin film transistor) detectors consist of arrays of semiconductor detectors, and another method uses a detector such as amorphous selenium or cesium iodide to capture the photons with amorphous silicon plates to amplify the signal produced.

Digital and computed radiology techniques are being used increasingly in clinical departments, with a consequent reduction in the use of photographic film.

Fluoroscopy – image intensifier

Image intensifiers use a fluoroscopic tube to form an image. The input screen is covered with a material that emits light photons when hit by X-ray photons. These are then converted to electrons, focused using an electron lens and accelerated towards an anode where they strike an output phosphor producing light, that is then viewed by a video camera and transmitted to viewing screen or film exposure system. Fluoroscopy allows real-time visualization of moving anatomic structures and monitoring of radiological procedures such as barium studies and angiography.

Advantages and limitations of plain X-ray

Plain radiography is readily available in the hospital setting and is frequently the first line of imaging investigation. It has a higher spatial resolution than all other imaging modalities. It is most useful for structures with high-density contrasts between tissue types, particularly those tissues in which fine detail is important, such as in viewing bone, and in the chest. Plain radiography is relatively poor for examining soft tissues, due to its limited contrast resolution. It is possible to distinguish only four natural densities in diagnostic radiography: calcium (bone), water (soft tissue), fat, and air. Plain film radiography provides a two-dimensional representation of three-dimensional structures; all structures projected in a direct line between the X-ray tube and the image receptor will overlap. This can be partially overcome by obtaining views from different angles, or by turning the patient or the X-ray tube and image intensifier in fluoroscopy.

Conventional tomography

Simultaneously moving both the X-ray tube and the film about a pivot point causes blurring of structures above and below the focal plane. Objects within the focal plane show increased detail because of the blurring of surrounding structures, providing an image of a slice of the patient (Fig. 1.6). Movements of the X-ray tube and film can be linear, elliptical, spiral, or hypocycloidal. With the advent of cross-sectional imaging techniques such as CT and MRI, most imaging departments now only use linear tomography, as part of an intravenous urogram (see below).

Contrast enhancing agents

To allow visualization of specific structures using X-rays, a number of contrast agents have been used. A good contrast agent should increase contrast resolution of organs under examination without poisoning or otherwise damaging the patient. The best contrast agents for use with X-rays have a high atomic weight as these have a high proportion of photoelectric absorption in the diagnostic X-ray range. Unfortunately, most molecules that contain these atoms are very toxic. Iodine (atomic weight 127) is the only element that has proved satisfactory for general intravascular use; extensive research and development has resulted in complex iodinated molecules that are non-toxic, hypoallergenic and do not carry too great osmotic load. The normal physiological turnover of iodine in the body is 0.0001 g per day, while for typical imaging applications 15 g to 150 g or 150 000–1 500 000 times as much may be required. Barium sulphate (atomic weight 137), and iodinated compounds are the only agents in regular use as extravascular agents.

Barium studies

Barium is only used in a modern X-ray department for studies of the gastrointestinal tract. These are usually based on a fluoroscopic image intensifier on which a moving image can be seen. Studies can be performed of the swallowing mechanism and esophagus (barium swallow), the stomach and duodenum (barium meal), the small bowel (small bowel follow through or small bowel enema) and the colon (barium enema). Studies of the stomach and large bowel are usually "double contrast" which allows better visualization of surface detail. Air or carbon dioxide can be introduced into the large bowel and gas-forming granules (usually a combination of calcium carbonate and citric acid) can be swallowed for imaging the stomach, resulting in a thin barium coating of the bowel mucosa (Fig. 1.7).

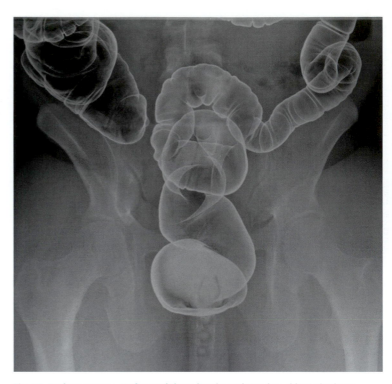

Fig. 1.7. **Barium enema. Barium sulphate has been introduced into the large bowel by a tube placed in the rectum and carbon dioxide gas is then used to expand the bowel, leaving a thin coating of barium on its inside surface. X-ray images are used to examine the lining of the bowel for abnormal growths and other abnormalities.**

Intravenous urography

The kidneys rapidly excrete Iodinated contrast agents. Plain radiographs taken from just a few seconds after a contrast injection into a peripheral vein show the passage of contrast through the kidney, into the ureters and to the bladder (Fig. 1.8).

Angiography

A specially shaped, thin catheter (tube) can be introduced into the arterial or venous system and manipulated using fluoroscopy to almost any blood vessel large enough to have been named. Contrast introduced through these catheters by hand or mechanical injection will be carried in the bloodstream and allows very detailed imaging of the vascular system. The arterial system is usually accessed via puncture of the femoral artery in the groin, although arteries of the upper limb may occasionally be used. Digital subtraction angiography (DSA) is most commonly performed – an initial ("mask") image is taken before the contrast agent is administered and is "subtracted" from later images. This removes the image of the tissues, leaving the contrast-filled structures. Any movement after the mask image is taken destroys the subtracted image. Because angiography is potentially hazardous, the balance between the potential benefit and the risk of the procedure (damage to vessels and other structures, bleeding) must be evaluated with particular care before undertaking the procedure (Fig. 1.9).

Radiation dose

All ionizing radiation exposure is associated with a small risk. A small proportion of the genetic mutations and cancers occurring in the population can be attributed to natural background radiation. Diagnostic

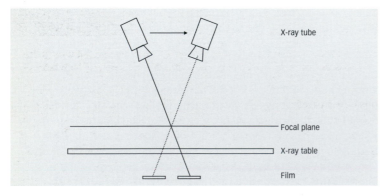

Fig. 1.6. **Conventional tomography. The X-ray tube and film move simultaneously about a pivot point at the level of the focal plane, blurring structures outside the focal plane, and emphasizing the structure of interest.**

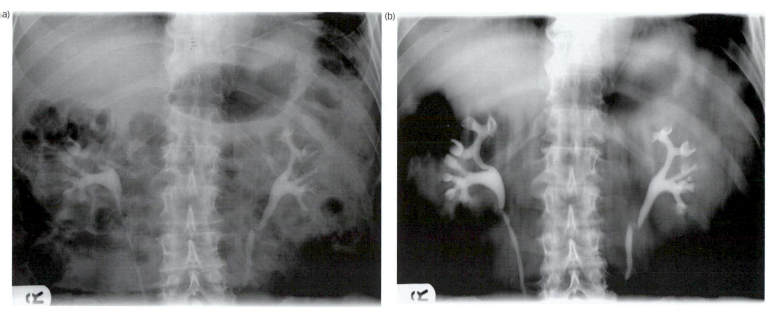

Fig. 1.8. **Intravenous urogram showing (a) standard view of the kidneys and upper part of the urinary collecting system and (b) linear tomogram of the intrarenal collecting system. This blurs out the overlying structures, giving a clearer image of the collecting system and renal outline. An injection of 50 ml of iodine-based contrast medium has been given and these radiographs have been obtained 10–15 minutes later after it has passed through the kidneys and into the renal collecting system.**

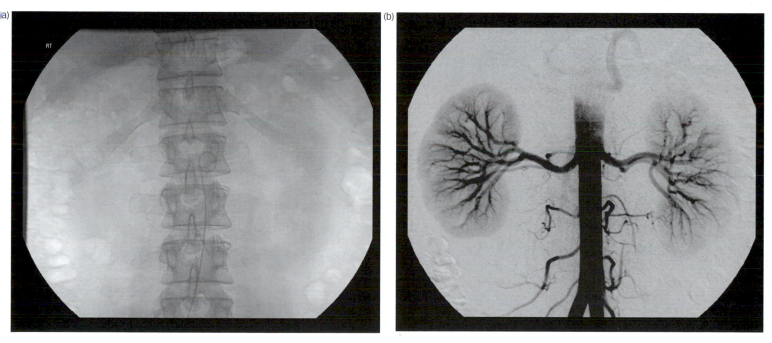

Fig. 1.9. **Renal angiogram. (a) A catheter has been inserted through the right femoral artery into the aorta, (b) iodinated contrast medium has been injected through it, and a rapid sequence of radiographs taken. Digital subtraction of the background shows the passage of contrast medium through the arteries supplying both kidneys.**

medical exposures (using X-rays or γ-rays, see Nuclear Medicine below) are the largest source of man-made radiation exposure to the general population and add about one-sixth to the population dose from background radiation. The dose is calculated as "effective dose," which is a weighted figure depending on the sensitivity of the body tissues involved to radiation induced cancer or genetic effects. Typical doses are given in Fig. 1.10. Children and the developing fetus are particularly susceptible to radiation damage. As with all medical investigations and procedures, the relative risks and potential benefits must be considered carefully, and the clinician directing the procedure (usually the radiologist) is accountable in law for any radiation exposure.

Ultrasound

General principles

Ultrasound is sound of very high frequency. In most diagnostic applications frequencies between two million and twenty million cycles per second are used, 100–1000 times higher than audible sound.

Procedure	Typical effective dose (mSv)	Equivalent number of chest X-rays	Equivalent period of natural background radiation
Limbs and joints	<0.01	<0.5	<1.5 days
Chest	0.02	1	3 days
Lumbar spine	1.3	65	7 months
Pelvis	0.7	35	4 months
Abdomen	1.0	50	6 months
IVU	2.5	125	14 months
Barium enema	7	350	3.2 years
CT head	2.3	115	1 year
CT chest	8	400	3.6 years
CT abdomen or pelvis	10	500	4.5 years
Bone scan	4	200	1.8 years
PET head (FDG)	5	250	2.3 years

Fig. 1.10. **Typical effective doses for some of the commonly performed imaging investigations. The typical United Kingdom background radiation dose is 2.2 mSv/year (ranges from 1.5 to 7.5 mSv/year depending on geographical location). It has been estimated that the additional lifetime risk of a fatal cancer from an abdominal CT scan could be as much as 1 in 2000 (although the overall lifetime risk of cancer for the whole population is 1 in 3).**

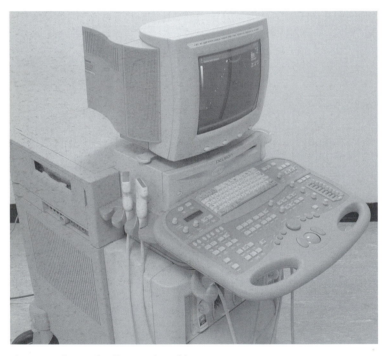

Fig. 1.11. **A diagnostic ultrasound machine.**

Higher frequencies have shorter wavelengths, allowing greater spatial resolution of structures being studied. An example of an ultrasound machine is shown in Fig. 1.11.

Ultrasound transducers
Ultrasound is generated by piezoelectric materials, such as lead zirconate titanate (PZT). These have the property of changing in thickness when a voltage is applied across them. When an electrical pulse is applied, the piezoelectric crystal produces sound at its resonant frequency. These crystals also generate a voltage when struck by an

ultrasound wave, so are also used as the receiver. A modern ultrasound probe contains an array of several hundred tiny piezoelectric crystals with metal electrodes on their two surfaces, the sound lenses and matching layers required to form the beam shape and electronics. Piezoelectric crystals can also be found in the speakers inside in-ear headsets, quartz watches, and camera auto-focus mechanisms.

Image formation
Ultrasound travels at near constant speed in soft tissues and this allows the depth of reflectors to be calculated by measuring the delay between transmission of the pulse and return of the echoes.

Attenuation
The tissues absorb ultrasound when the orderly vibration of the sound wave becomes disordered in the presence of large molecules. When this happens, sound energy is converted to heat energy. Absorption depends on the molecular size, which correlates with viscosity of the tissue, and with the frequency. Higher frequencies are more strongly absorbed, so less depth of scanning comes with the improvement in resolution that higher frequencies allow. Ultrasound energy is also lost to the transducer if it is reflected or refracted away.

Reflection
Some of the ultrasound beam is reflected whenever it crosses an interface where the transmission properties change. This is directly related to the physical structure of the tissues on either side of the interface.

Tissue harmonics
Ultrasound is generally considered to be conducted in a linear fashion with no change in the waveform of the pulse as it travels through the tissues. In fact, the wave originating from the transducer becomes distorted as the speed of sound conduction changes with the density of the conducting materials allowing some parts of the wave to travel faster than others. The wave comes to contain higher frequency components, called harmonics, which are much weaker in the parts of the sound beam away from the central echoes. Scanners can transmit at one frequency, receive at a higher frequency and use filters to select out the harmonics in the returning echoes, improving the image resolution and increasing the contrast.

Image display
Gray-scale or B-Mode (B for brightness) is a two-dimensional real time image formed by sweeping the beam through the tissue. The echogenicity of the reflectors is displayed as shades of gray and is the main mode used for ultrasound imaging (Fig. 1.12). Modern ultrasound machines operate at a sufficient speed to produce real-time images of moving patient tissue such as the heart in echocardiography and the moving fetus.

Doppler ultrasound
If a sound wave reflects from a moving target, there is a change in the frequency of the returning sound wave proportional to the velocity of the reflecting target. This is known as the Doppler effect and the changes in frequency can be used to calculate the velocity of the moving target usually flowing blood. The Doppler signal is within the audible range, so can be heard by sending the signal to a loudspeaker. Most commonly used in clinical practice is color flow imaging (color Doppler) where flow information is shown as an overlay on the gray-scale image with the color and shading indicating the direction

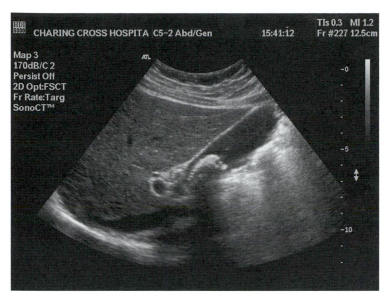

Fig. 1.12. **A stone within the gall bladder shows as a bright echo with black "acoustic shadow" behind it, the result of almost complete reflection of the ultrasound hitting it. The fluid in the gall bladder appears black as the contents of the gall bladder are homogeneous and there are no internal structures to cause echoes or changes in attenuation; the adjacent liver is more complex in structure and causes more reflection of sound, so appears gray.**

and velocity of flow. Spectral Doppler is a graphical display with time on the horizontal axis, frequency on the vertical axis and brightness of the tracing indicating the number of echoes at each specific frequency (and therefore blood cell velocity). A combined gray-scale and spectral Doppler display is known as a duplex scan. Power Doppler imaging discards the direction and velocity information but is about 10× more sensitive to flow than normal color Doppler.

Doppler ultrasound is used to image blood vessels and to examine tissues for vascularity (fig. 1.13 – see color plate section).

Ultrasound contrast agents

Contrast agents have been developed for ultrasound consisting of tiny "microbubbles" of gas small enough to cross the capillary bed of the lungs. These are safe for injection into the bloodstream and are very highly reflective; they can be used to improve the imaging of blood vessels and to examine the filling patterns of liver lesions.

Ultrasound artifacts
Acoustic shadowing

Produced by near complete absorption or reflection of the ultrasound beam, obscuring deeper structures. Acoustic shadows are produced by bone, calcified structures (such as gall bladder and kidney stones), gas in bowel, and metallic structures.

Acoustic enhancement

Structures that transmit sound well such as fluid-filled structures (bladder, cysts) cause an increased intensity of echoes deep to the structure.

Reverberation artifact

Repeated, bouncing echoes between strong acoustic reflectors cause multiple echoes from the same structure, shown as repeating bands of echoes at regularly spaced intervals.

Mirror image artifact

A strong reflector can cause duplication of echoes, giving the appearance of duplication of structures above and below the reflector.

"Ring down" artifact

A pattern of tapering bright echoes trailing from small bright reflectors such as air bubbles.

Advantages and limitations of ultrasound

Ultrasound provides images in real time so can be used to image movement of structures such as heart valves and patterns of blood flow within vessels. As far as is known, ultrasound used at diagnostic intensities does not cause tissue damage and can be used to image sensitive structures such as the developing fetus. Patients usually find ultrasound examination easy to tolerate, as it requires minimal preparation and only light pressure on the skin. Portable ultrasound systems suitable for use at the bedside are widely available.

The main limitation of the technique is that parts of the body accessible to ultrasound examination are limited. Ultrasound does not easily cross a tissue–gas or tissue–bone interface, so can only be used for imaging tissues around such structures with any tissues deep to gas or bone obscured. It is not generally useful in the lungs and head, except in neonates where the open fontanelles provide an acoustic window. Ultrasound is also heavily operator dependent, particularly in overcoming barriers due to the bony skeleton and bowel gas, and in interpreting artifacts, which are common.

Computed tomography

Computed tomography (CT) was invented in the 1970s, earning its chief inventor, Sir Godfrey Hounsfield, the Nobel Prize for medicine in 1979. CT was the first fully digital imaging technique that provided cross-sectional images of any anatomical structure.

Basic principles

Current generation CT scanners use the same basic technology as the first clinical EMI machine in 1972. In conventional CT, the X-ray tube and detector rotate around the patient with the table stationary. The X-ray beam is attenuated by absorption and scatter as it passes through the patient with the detector measuring transmission (fig. 1.14). Multiple measurements are taken from different directions as the tube and detector rotate. A computer reconstructs the image for this single "slice." The patient and table are then moved to the next slice position and the next image is obtained.

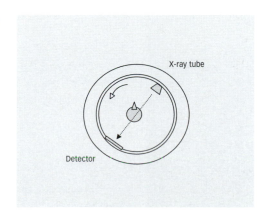

Fig. 1.14. **Diagram of a typical CT scanner. The patient is placed on the couch and the X-ray tube rotates 360° around the patient, producing pulses of radiation that pass through the patient. The detectors rotate with the tube, on the other side of the patient detect the attenuated X-ray pulse. This data is sent to a computer for reconstruction.**

In spiral (helical) CT the X-ray tube rotates continuously while the patient and table move through the scanner. Instead of obtaining data as individual slices, a block of data in the form of a helix is obtained. Scans can be performed during a single breath hold, which reduces misregistration artifacts, such as occur when a patient has a different depth of inspiration between conventional scans. A typical CT scanner is shown in Fig. 1.15.

Image reconstruction

To convert the vast amount of raw data obtained during scanning to the image requires mathematical transformation. Depending on the parameters used (known as "kernels"), it is possible to get either a high spatial resolution (at the expense of higher noise levels) used for lung and bone imaging, or a high signal to noise ratio (at the expense of lower resolution) used for soft tissues.

The CT image consists of a matrix of image elements (pixels) usually 256×256 or 512×512 pixels. Each of these displays a gray scale intensity value representing the X-ray attenuation of the corresponding block of tissue, known as a voxel (a three-dimensional "volume element").

CT scanners operate at relatively high diagnostic X-ray energies, in the order of 100 kV. At these energies, the majority of X-ray-tissue interactions are by Compton scatter, so the attenuation of the X-ray beam is directly proportional to the density of the tissues. The intensity value is scored in Hounsfield units (HU). By definition, water is 0 HU and air −1000 HU and the values are assigned proportionately. These values can be used to differentiate between tissue types. Air (−1000 HU) and fat (−100 HU) have negative values, most soft tissues have values just higher than water (0 HU), e.g., muscle (30 HU), liver (60 HU), while bone and calcified structures have values of 200–900 HU. The contrast resolution of CT depends on the differences between these values, the larger the better. Although better than plain X-ray in differentiating soft tissue types, CT is not a good as magnetic resonance imaging (MRI). For applications in the lungs and bone (where the differences in attenuation values are large), CT is generally better than MRI.

The use of intravenous contrast agents can increase the contrast resolution in soft tissues as different tissues show differences in enhancement patterns. Oral contrast can outline the lumen of bowel and allow differentiation of bowel contents and soft tissues within the abdomen. Usually iodinated contrast agents are used for CT, although a dilute barium solution can be used as bowel contrast.

Window and level

The human eye cannot appreciate anywhere near the 4000 or so gray scale values obtained in a single CT slice. If the full range of reconstructed values were all displayed so as to cover all perceived brightness values uniformly, a great deal of information would be lost as the viewer would not be able to distinguish the tiny differences between differing HU values. By restricting the range of gray scale information displayed, more subtle variations in intensity can be shown. This is done by varying the range ("window width") and centre ("window level") (Fig. 1.16).

Spiral CT and pitch

In conventional, incremental CT the parameters describing the procedure are slice width and table increment (the movement of the table between slices). With spiral CT, the patient, lying on the couch, moves into the scanner as the tube and detectors rotate in a continuous movement, rather than the couch remaining still while each "slice" is acquired. The information during spiral CT is obtained as a continuous stream and is reconstructed into slices.

The parameters for spiral CT are slice collimation (the width of the X-ray beam and therefore the amount of the patient covered per rotation), table feed per rotation, and the reconstruction increment. A spiral CT covers the whole volume even if the table feed is greater than the collimation – it is possible to scan with a table feed up to twice the collimation without major loss of image quality. Often, scans are described by their pitch where pitch = table feed/collimation. Typical values for collimation (slice thickness) are 1–10 mm with rotation times of 0.5–3 seconds.

To reconstruct from the helical volume, it is necessary to interpolate the projections of one scanner rotation. It is not necessary to reconstruct as consecutive slices – slices with any amount of overlap can be created.

Multi-detector CT

CT scanners are now available with multiple rows of detectors (at the time of writing, commonly 64) allowing acquisition of multiple slices in one spiral acquisition. In conjunction with fast rotation speeds, the volume coverage and speed performance are improved allowing, for instance, an abdomen and pelvis to be scanned with an acquisition slice thickness of 1.25 mm in about quarter the time (approximately 10 seconds) that a 10 mm collimation CT scanner could cover the same volume, with the same or lesser radiation dose. The main problem with this type of scanning is the number of images acquired; 300–400 in the example above instead of about 40 with single slice techniques.

Advanced image reconstructions

From the spiral dataset, further reconstructions can be performed. Multiplanar reformats (MPR) can be performed in any selected plane, although usually in the coronal and sagittal planes (Fig. 1.17). Three-dimensional reconstructions can also be obtained using techniques

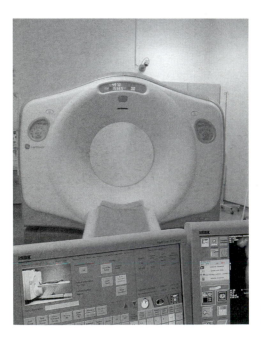

Fig. 1.15. **A multi-slice CT scanner.**

(a)

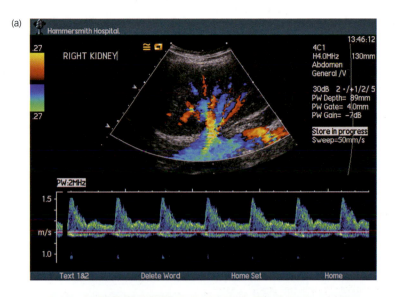

(b)

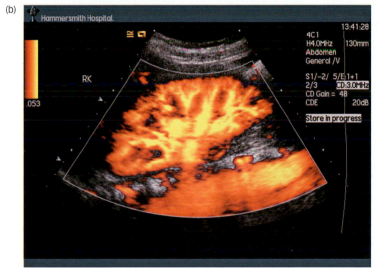

Fig. 1.13. **(a) Color (top) and spectral Doppler (bottom) and (b) power Doppler ultrasound images of a right kidney showing the blood vessels within it. The color Doppler shows the direction of the blood with blood moving towards the probe (the top of the image) shown as red and blood moving away from the image shown as blue. The spectral Doppler shows the waveform of the blood within the renal artery.**

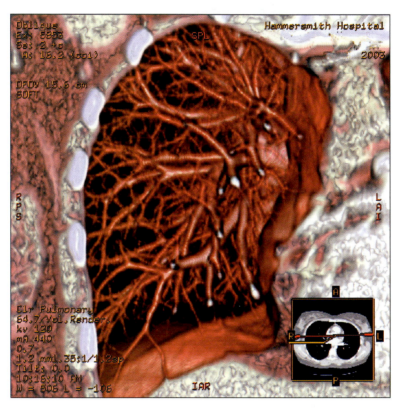

Fig. 1.18. **An example of volume rendering showing blood vessels within the lung of the same subject as Figs. 16 and 17. While providing an attractive image, this contains less diagnostic information than the whole scan when viewed using the projections in the other two figures.**

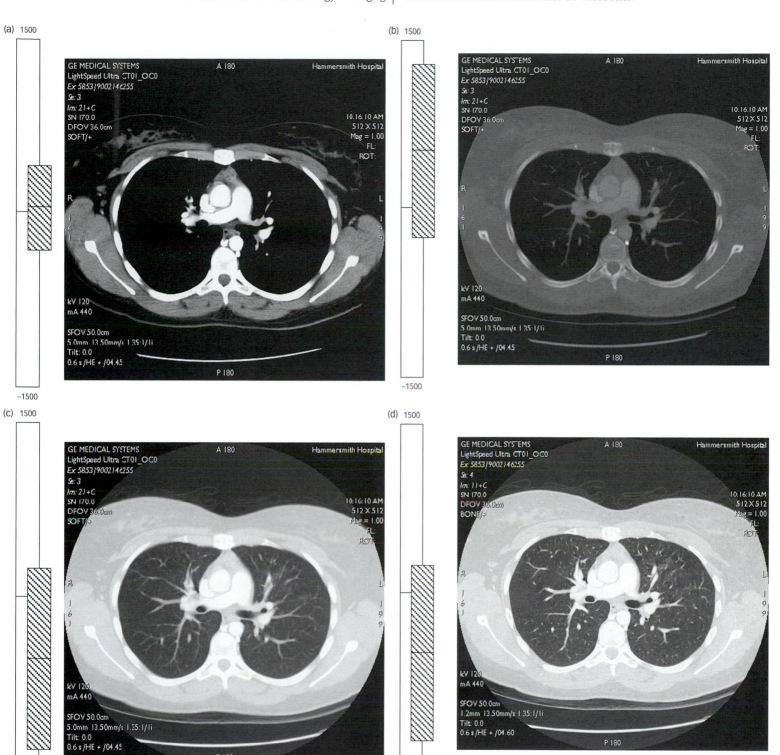

Fig. 1.16. **The effect of changing window levels and reconstruction algorithm on a single axial image through the chest. The dark bar indicated the range of values displayed, the light bar the range of values available. (a) "Soft tissue" window with window level of 350 and centre 50; (b) "bone window" with window level 1500 and centre 500; (c) lung window with window level 1500 and centre −500; and (d) an HRCT (high resolution CT image) – this is a thin slice image reconstructed using an edge enhancement (bone or lung) algorithm, which shows better detail in the lung but increases "noise" levels, window 1500, centre −500.**

such as surface-shaded display and volume rendering (Fig. 1.18 – see color plate section). While the 3-D techniques provide attractive images and are useful in giving an overview of complex anatomical structures, a lot of information from the original axial data set is often discarded. Virtual endoscopy uses a 3-D "central" projection to give the effect of viewing a hollow viscus interiorly (as is seen in endoscopic examination) and is of particular use in patients too frail or ill to have invasive endoscopy.

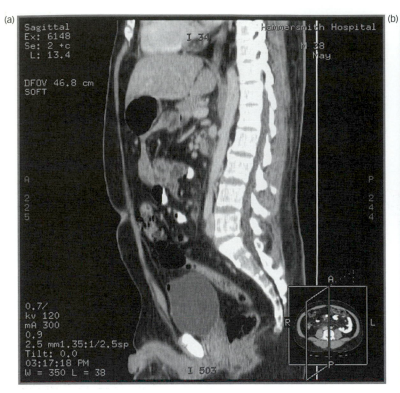

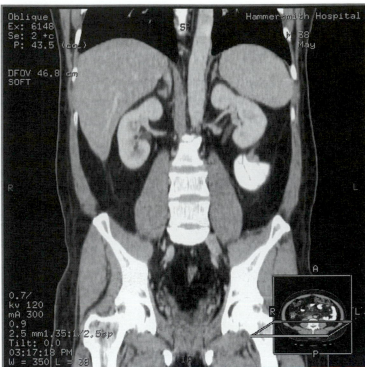

Fig. 1.17. **(a) Sagittal** and **(b) coronal** reformats of a helical scan through the abdomen and pelvis. The data from the axial slices is rearranged to give different projections.

HRCT

High resolution CT or HRCT is used to image the lungs. Thin slices are acquired – usually 1 to 2 mm thick at 10–20 mm intervals. These are reconstructed using edge enhancement (bone or lung) algorithms showing better detail in the lung but increasing "noise" levels (Fig. 1.16). This allows fine details of lung anatomy to be seen. The whole lung volume is not scanned, as there are gaps between the slices.

CT artifacts
Volume averaging

A single CT slice of 10 mm thickness can contain more than one tissue type within each voxel (for example, bone and lung). The CT number for that voxel will be an average of the different sorts of tissue within it, so very small structures can be "averaged out" or if a structure with low CT number is adjacent to one with a high CT number, the apparent tissue density will be somewhere in between. This is known as a "partial volume effect."

Beam hardening artifact

This results from greater attenuation of low-energy photons than high-energy photons as the beam passes through the tissue. The average energy of the X-ray beam increases so there is less attenuation at the end of the beam than at the beginning, giving streaks of low density extending from areas of high density such as bones.

Motion artifact

This occurs when there is movement of structures during image acquisition and shows up as blurred or duplicated images, or as streaking.

Streak artifact

The reconstruction algorithms cannot deal with the differences in X-ray attenuation between very high-density objects such as metal clips or fillings in the teeth and the adjacent tissues and produce high attenuation streaks running from the dense object (Fig. 1.19).

Advantages and limitations of CT

CT provides a rapid, non-invasive method of assessing patients. A whole body scan can be performed in a few seconds on a modern multislice scanner with very good anatomical detail. CT is particularly suited to high X-ray contrast structures such as the bones and the lungs, and remains the cross-sectional imaging modality of choice for assessing these. It has less contrast resolution than MRI for soft tissue structures particularly for intracranial imaging, spinal imaging, and musculoskeletal imaging. CT has no major contraindications (although the use of contrast might have), providing the patient can tolerate the scan. The major disadvantage is in the significant radiation doses required for CT. An abdominal or pelvic CT involves 3–12 mSv of radiation, compared with a chest X-ray's 0.02 mSv or background radiation in the UK averaging 2.5 mSv per year.

Magnetic resonance imaging (MRI)

Nuclear magnetic resonance was first described in 1946 as a tool for determining molecular structure. The ability to produce an image based on the distribution of hydrogen nuclei within a sample, the basis of the modern MRI scanner, was first described in 1973 and the first commercial body scanner was launched in 1978. A modern MRI scanner is shown in Fig. 1.20.

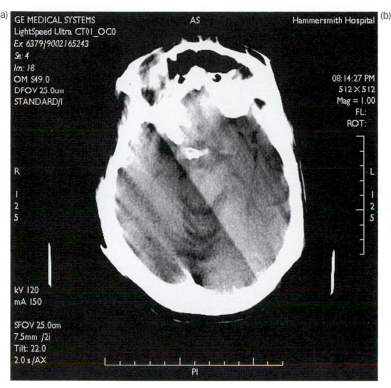

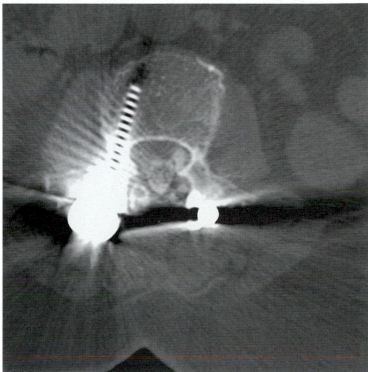

Fig. 1.19. **(a) Movement artifact in a CT head scan. There is blurring and streaking following movement of the head. (b) Streak artifact from screws and rods used to immobilize the lumbar spine.**

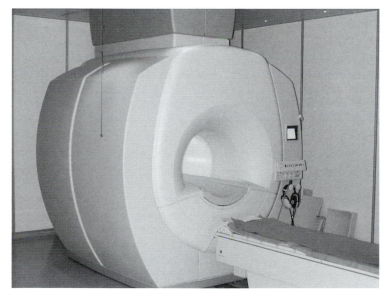

Fig. 1.20. **A magnetic resonance (MR) scanner.**

Basic principles

Detailed explanation of the complicated physics of MRI is beyond the scope of this chapter. More detailed descriptions of MRI, using a relatively accessible and non-mathematical approach, may be found in the recommended texts for further reading below.

MRI involves the use of magnetic fields and radio waves to produce tomographic images. Normal clinical applications involve the imaging of hydrogen nuclei (protons) only, although other atoms possessing a "net magnetic moment," such as phosphorus 31, can also be used. As most protons in biological tissues are in water, clinical MRI is mainly about imaging water.

The protons in the patient's tissues can be thought of as containing tiny bar magnets, which are normally randomly oriented in space.

The patient is placed within a strong magnetic field, which causes a small proportion (about two per million) of the atomic nuclei to align in the direction of the field and spin (precess) at a specific frequency. Current magnets typically use a 1.5 tesla field, about 30 000 times the earth's natural magnetic field. When radio waves (radio frequency, RF) are applied at the specific (resonance) frequency, energy is absorbed by the nuclei, causing them all to precess together, and causing some to flip their orientation. When the transmitter is turned off, these flip back to their equilibrium position, stop precessing together and emit radiowaves, which are detectable by an aerial and amplified electronically. The frequency of resonance is proportional to the magnetic field that the proton experiences.

The signal is localized in the patient by the use of smaller magnetic field gradients across and along the patient (in all three planes). These cause a predictable variation in the magnetic field strength and in the resonant frequency in different parts of the patient. By varying the times at which the gradient fields are switched on in relation to applying radio frequency pulses, and by analysis of the frequency and phase information of the emitted radio signal, a computer is able to construct a three-dimensional image of the patient.

The proton relaxes to a lower energy state by two main processes, called longitudinal recovery (which has a recovery time, T_1) and transverse relaxation (with a relaxation time, T_2), and re-emits its energy as radiowaves. The relative proportions of T_1 and T_2 vary between different tissues.

(a)

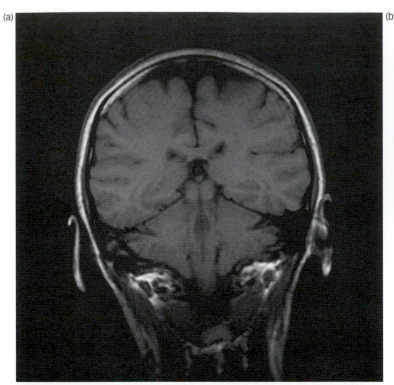

(b)

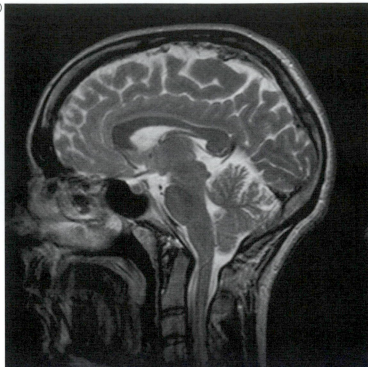

(c)

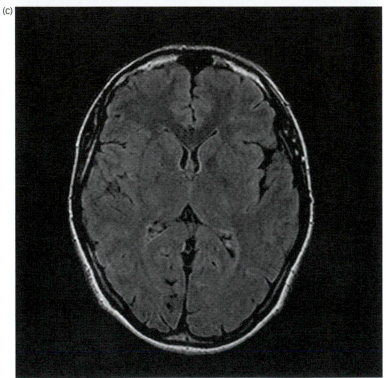

Fig. 1.21. **(a) Coronal T1W, (b) sagittal T2W and (c) axial FLAIR** slices through the brain. Cerebrospinal fluid is low signal (black) on the T1W and FLAIR images but high signal (white) on the T2W image.

T1 times are long in water and shorten when larger molecules are present so cerebrospinal fluid (which is largely water) has a T1 time of about 1500 milliseconds, while muscle (which has water bound to proteins) has a T1 time of 500 milliseconds and fat (which has its own protons, much more tightly bound than those in water) has a very

short T1 time of about 230 ms. T2 relaxation times largely depends on tiny local variations in magnetic field due to the presence of neighbouring nuclei. In pure water, T2 times are long (similar to T1 times); in solid structures there is very much more effect from the neighbouring nuclei and T2 times can be only a few milliseconds.

By altering the pulse sequence and scanning parameters, one or other process can be emphasized, hence T1 weighted (T1W) scans where signal intensity is most sensitive to changes in T1, and T2 weighted (T2W) scans where signal intensity is most sensitive to changes in T2. This allows signal contrast between different normal tissue types to be optimized, such as gray and white matter and cerebrospinal fluid in the brain, and pathological foci to be accentuated.

There are a number of ways in which the magnetic field gradients and RF pulses can be used to generate different types of MR images

T1 and T2 weighting and proton density

Standard spin echo sequences produce standard T1 weighted (T1W), T2 weighted (T2W) and proton density (PD) scans. T1W scans traditionally provide the best anatomic detail. T2W scans usually provide the most sensitive detection of pathology. Proton density-weighted images make T1 and T2 relaxation times less important and instead provide information about the density of protons within the tissue.

In the brain, cerebrospinal fluid (mainly water) is dark on T1W scans and bright on T2W scans (Fig. 1.21).

Inversion recovery (IR) sequences

These sequences emphasize differences in T1 relaxation times of tissues. The MR operator selects a delay time, called the inversion time, which is added to the TR and TE settings. Short tau (T1) inversion time (STIR) sequences are the most commonly used and suppress the signal from fat while emphasizing tissues with high water content as high signal, including most areas of pathology. Fluid attenuated inversion-recovery (FLAIR) sequences have a longer inversion time and

(a)
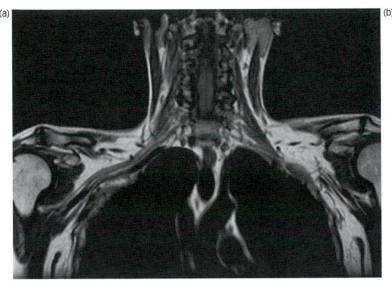
(b)
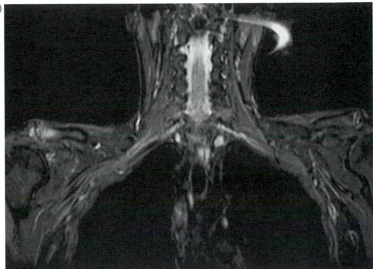

Fig. 1.22. **MR images of the upper part of the thorax showing the brachial plexus, demonstrating the effects of fat suppression. On the T1W sequence (a), the fat is high signal (white) and on the STIR sequence (b) the signal from fat is reduced.**

are used to image the brain as they null the signal from cerebrospinal fluid, improving conspicuity of pathology in adjacent structures. FLAIR images are mostly T2 weighted but CSF looks darker (Fig. 1.21).

Turbo (fast) spin echo and echo-planar imaging

These are faster MR techniques that produce multiple slices in shorter times. There is an image quality penalty to be paid for faster acquisitions and artifacts may manifest differently.

Gradient recalled echo or gradient echo sequences

Gradient echo (GE or GRE) sequences use gradient field changes rather than RF pulse sequences. Gradient echo sequences can be T1W or T2W, although the T2W images are actually T2* ("T2 star"), which is a less "pure" form of T2 weighting than in spin echo. Artifacts tend to be more prominent in gradient techniques, particularly those due to local disturbances of the magnetic field because of the presence of tissue interfaces and metal (including iron in blood degradation products).

Fat suppression

Fat-containing tissues have high signal on both T1W and T2W scans. This can overwhelm the signal from adjacent structures of more interest, so MR sequences have been developed to reduce the signal from fat. The STIR sequence described above is one of these. Fat saturation is another technique that can be used in which a presaturation RF pulse tuned to the resonant frequency of fat protons is applied to the tissues before the main pulse sequence, causing a nulling of the signal from the fatty tissues (Fig. 1.22).

Diffusion-weighted imaging (DWI)

Changes in the diffusion of tissue water can be visualized using this technique, which relies on small random movements of the molecules changing the distribution of phases. This technique is used to image pathology within the brain, particularly early ischemic strokes.

MR angiography

MR angiograms often use a "time of flight" sequence where the inflowing blood is saturated with a preliminary RF pulse sequence,

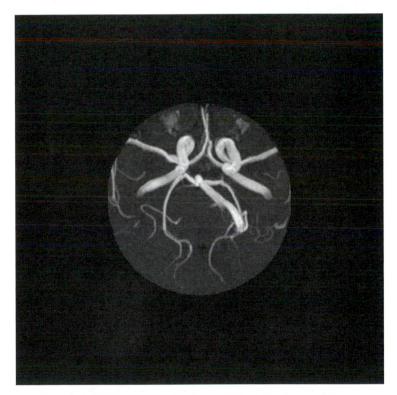

Fig. 1.23. **A single MIP (maximum intensity projection) view from an MR angiogram showing the large vessels of the intracerebral circulation. This angiogram has been created from a time-of-flight (TOF) scanning sequence.**

or use MR contrast agents. In these, flowing blood in vessels is of high signal. A MR angiogram is usually viewed as a maximum intensity projection or MIP (Fig. 1.23). To create an MIP, only the high signal structures are shown and all the MR slices are compressed together (or projected) to give a single view as if looking at the subject from a particular angle. Usually, projections from multiple angles are used. Other methods relying on phase contrast or injected intravascular contrast media may also be used.

(a)

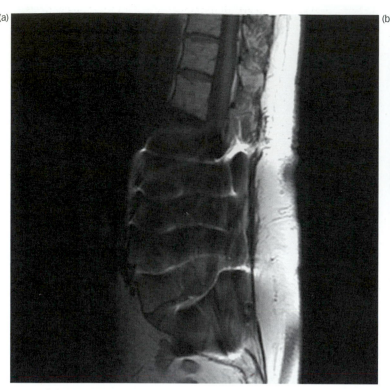

(b)

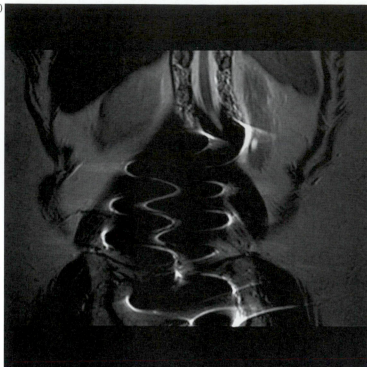

Fig. 1.24. **(a) Sagittal T1W and b) coronal T2W** images from an MR examination of the spine in a patient who has had surgery with metal screws and rods along the lower spine. There is marked loss of signal and distortion of the surrounding structures over most of the scan.

Magnetic resonance cholangiopancreaticogram

MRCP or magnetic resonance cholangiopancreaticography images are used to image the biliary system non-invasively, and are created as a MIP of a sequence in which fluid is of high signal.

MR artifacts

Ferromagnetic artifact

All ferromagnetic objects, such as orthopedic implants, surgical clips and wire, dental fillings, and metallic foreign bodies cause major distortions in the main magnetic field, giving areas of signal void and distortion (Fig. 1.24). Even tattoos and mascara can contain enough ferromagnetic pigments to cause a significant reduction in image quality.

Susceptibility artifact

This is due to local changes in the field from to the differing magnetisation of tissue types, rather like a less pronounced form of ferromagnetic artifact. Susceptibility artifacts usually occur at interfaces between other tissue types and bone or air-filled structures.

Motion artifact

The acquisition time for MR is relatively lengthy and image degradation due to movement artifacts is common. General movement, including breathing, causes blurring of the image. Pulsation from blood vessels causes ghosts of the moving structures (Fig. 1.25)

Chemical shift artifact

This occurs at interfaces between fat and water. Protons in fat have a slightly different resonance frequency compared with those in water, which can lead to a misregistration of their location. This gives a high signal–low signal line on either side of the interface.

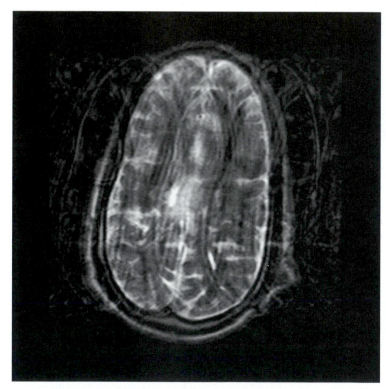

Fig. 1.25. **Axial T$_2$W image of the brain in a patient unable to lie sufficiently still.**

Aliasing (wraparound) artifact

This can occur when part of the anatomy outside the field of view of the scan is incorrectly placed within the image, on the opposite side. This occurs in the phase encoding direction and can be removed by increasing the field of view (although at the expense of either resolution or time). It is common in echo planar imaging.

MRI safety

MR is contraindicated in patients with electrically, magnetically, or mechanically activated implants including cardiac pacemakers, cochlear implants, neurostimulators and insulin, and other implantable drug infusion pumps. Ferromagnetic implants such as cerebral aneurysm clips and surgical staples, and bullets, shrapnel, and metal fragments can move. Patients with a history of metallic foreign bodies in the eye should be screened with radiographs of the orbits.

A number of implants have been shown to be safe for MR including non-ferrous surgical clips and orthopedic devices made from non-ferrous metals. Contemporary devices are largely MRI compatible, although older ones may not be.

MR magnetic fields can induce electrical currents in conductors, such as in cables for monitoring equipment attached to the patient (e.g., ECG leads), with a risk of electric shock to the patient. Any monitor leads must be carefully designed and tested for MR compatibility to avoid this possibility.

There is no evidence that MR harms the developing fetus. Pregnant patients can be scanned, although as a precaution MR is not usually performed in the first 3 months of pregnancy.

Advantages of MR

MR allows outstanding soft tissue contrast resolution and allows images to be created in any plane. No ionizing radiation is involved. It gives limited detail in structures such as cortical bone and calcification, which return negligible signal. MR has long scanning times in relation to other techniques and requires patients to be stationary while the scan is performed. Because of long imaging times and complexity of the equipment, MR is relatively expensive. The space within the magnet is restricted (a long tunnel) and some patients experience claustrophobia and are unable to tolerate the scan. Access to medically unstable patients is hindered and special, MR compatible, monitoring equipment is required.

Nuclear medicine

Nuclear medicine involves the imaging of Gamma rays (γ-rays), a type of electromagnetic radiation. The difference between γ-rays and X-rays is that γ-rays are produced from within the nucleus of the atom when unstable nuclei undergo transition (decay) to a more stable state, while X-rays are produced by bombarding the atom with electrons. Nuclear medicine imaging therefore is emission imaging – the γ-rays are produced within the patient and the photons are emitted from the subject and then detected.

Radiopharmaceuticals

The γ-ray emitter must first be administered to the patient – the substance given is known as a radiopharmaceutical. These consist of either radioactive isotopes by themselves, or more commonly radioisotopes (usually called radionuclides) attached to some other molecule. Radionuclides can be created in nuclear reactors, in cyclotrons and from generators. The most commonly used radionuclide is Technetium 99 m (Tc-99 m), which is produced from a generator containing Molybdenum-99 that is first created in a nuclear reactor as a product of Uranium-235 fission. Isotopes of iodine, krypton, phosphorus, gallium, indium, chromium, cobalt, fluorine,

thallium, and strontium are all in regular use. Radiopharmaceuticals are normally administered by injection into the venous system but are also administered orally, directly into body cavities, and by injection into soft tissues.

The gamma camera

Standard nuclear medicine images are acquired using a gamma camera (Fig. 1.26). The basic detector in the gamma camera consists of a sodium iodide crystal that emits light photons when struck by a γ-ray, with photo-multiplier tubes to detect the light photons emitted. The photo-multiplier tube produces an electrical voltage that is converted by the electronic and computer circuitry to a "dot" on the final image. The build-up of dots gives the final image (Fig. 1.27). Between the patient and the detector is a collimator which consists of a large lead block with holes in it that select only photons travelling at right angles to the detector. Those passing at an angle do not contribute to the image.

Single photon emission computed tomography (SPECT)

Computed tomography (CT, described above) allows the reconstruction of a three dimensional image from multiple projections of an external X-ray beam. A similar effect can be obtained in nuclear medicine with reconstruction of emissions of radionuclide within the patient from different projections. This is usually achieved by rotating the gamma camera head around the patient.

SPECT has the advantage of improving image contrast by minimizing the image activity present from overlying structures in a two-dimensional acquisition and allows improved three-dimensional localization of radiopharmaceuticals.

Positron emission tomography (PET)

PET deals with the detection and imaging of positron emitting radionuclides. A positron is a negative electron, a tiny particle of antimatter. Positrons are emitted from the decay of proton rich radionuclides such as carbon-11, nitrogen-13, oxygen-15 and fluorine-18. When a positron is emitted, it travels a short distance (a few mm) before encountering an electron; the electron and positron are

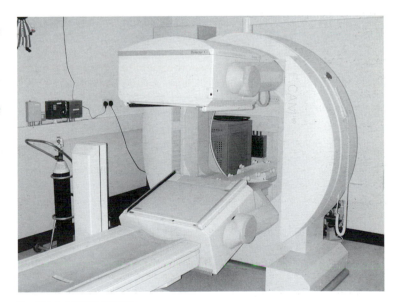

Fig. 1.26. **A gamma camera.**

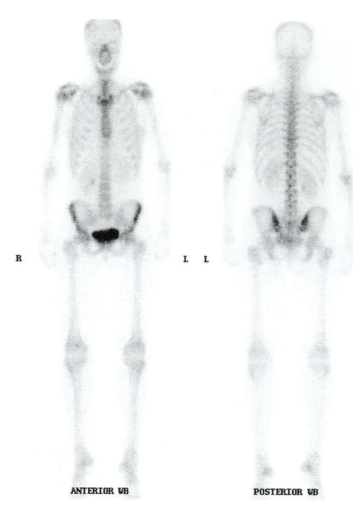

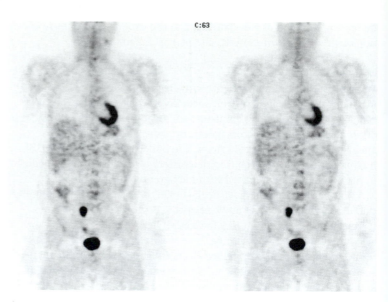

Fig. 1.28. **Coronal presentation of data from an FDG PET scan in a patient with lymphoma. A previously unrecognized site of disease within a right common iliac lymph node takes up the FDG and appears a an area of high uptake (black). Other normal, physiological sites of uptake include heart muscle, the liver and spleen, and the bones. Excretion is via the renal system, so the bladder also appears of high activity. (FDG = fluoro-deoxy-glucose; the glucose labelled with fluorine-18).**

Fig. 1.27. **A bone scan. Tc-99 m MDP, which is taken up by osteoblasts within bone, has been intravenously injected and an image acquired 3 hours later using a gamma camera. Uptake of the radionuclide can be seen within the bones, and also within the kidneys (faintly) and bladder – this radiopharmaceutical is excreted by the renal system.**

annihilated, releasing energy as two 511 keV γ-rays, which are emitted in opposite directions. The detectors in the PET scanner are set up in pairs and wait for a "coincidence" detection of two 511 keV γ-rays. A line drawn between the two detectors is then used in the computed tomography reconstruction (as in CT).

Most PET isotopes are made in cyclotrons and have very short half-lives (usually only a few minutes to hours). A commonly used PET chemical is FDG or fluoro-deoxy-glucose – glucose labelled with fluorine-18. Tissues that are actively metabolizing glucose take this up. PET has been particularly successful in imaging brain, heart, and oncological metabolism. PET scans generally have a higher resolution than SPECT scans (Fig. 1.28).

PET CT

Manufacturers have now combined PET and CT in a single scanner in which the PET image is coregistered with CT. This improves the anatomical accuracy of PET and is valuable in localizing disseminated disease, notably cancer.

PET CT is particularly helpful in recurrent cancers of the head and neck where post surgical change and scarring can mask new disease

Advantages of nuclear medicine

Isotope scans provide excellent physiological and functional information. They can often indicate the site of disease before there has been sufficient disruption of anatomy for it to be visible on other imaging techniques. Scans can be repeated over time to show the movement or uptake of radionuclide tracers. However, nuclear medicine studies sacrifice the high resolution of other imaging techniques. Isotope studies involve ionizing radiation, and for some longer half-life radioisotopes, patients can continue to emit low levels of ionizing radiation for several days. Some isotopes, particularly those used in PET scanning, are relatively expensive, and some isotopes for PET scanning are so short lived that an on-site cyclotron is required.

ADAM W. M. MITCHELL

In order to attempt to interpret a radiographic image, it is essential that you first identify the type of examination and understand something of the principles behind it. Before examining any image, the name of the patient and the date of the study should be checked. The film should also be hung correctly and right and left sides ascertained.

Plain radiography

Plain radiographs are the most commonly encountered of all imaging studies. The following chapters explain the radiological anatomy involved, but it is equally important to appreciate how the film was taken.

Staff in the radiology department can offer advice on any additional projections but it is very important from the outset to provide as much information as possible in the request for an examination, so that the correct views and exposures are used.

In general, over-exposed (dark), radiographs are more useful than those that are under-exposed, since the former retain the information. Rather than request another film and expose the patient to more ionizing radiation, the dark film should be examined with a bright light in the first instance.

Digital radiographs can be interrogated by "windowing" (see below), and although the original exposure must be correct, the resulting image can be manipulated to highlight bone or soft tissue detail as required.

The chest radiograph

The frontal chest radiograph is the most commonly requested plain film. The image is taken either as a "PA" (posteroanterior) or as an "AP" (anteroposterior), depending on the direction of the X-ray beam. The projection is usually marked on the film.

A PA projection is the better quality film and allows the size and shape of the heart and mediastinum to be assessed accurately. A PA film is taken with the patient erect and is performed in the radiology department. This, of course, requires the patient to be reasonably mobile (fig. 2.1).

For the less mobile or bed-bound patient, portable films are taken. These are all AP and can be taken with the patient supine or erect.

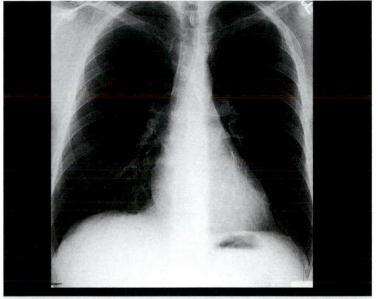

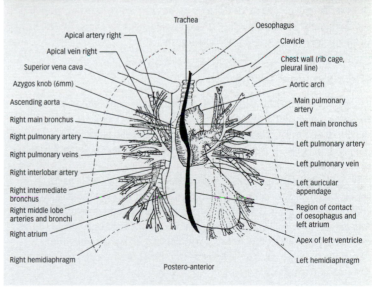

Fig. 2.1. **Normal PA chest radiograph.**

Applied Radiological Anatomy for Medical Students. Paul Butler, Adam Mitchell, and Harold Ellis (eds.) Published by Cambridge University Press. © P. Butler, A. Mitchell, and H. Ellis 2007.

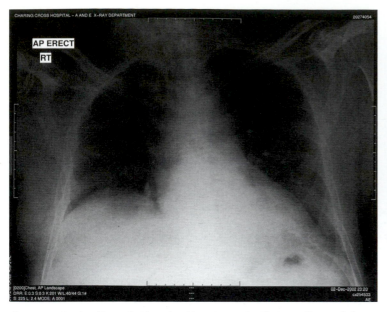

Fig. 2.2. **AP chest radiograph. There has been a poor respiratory effort and there is a false impression of cardiac enlargement.**

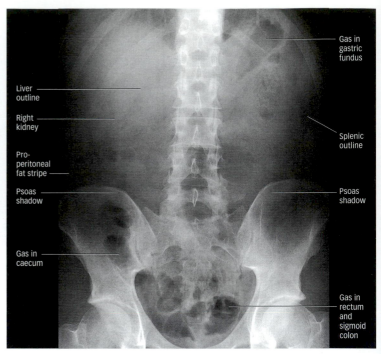

Fig. 2.3. **Plain abdominal radiograph.**

Because the divergent X-ray beam causes magnification, AP films can give a false impression of cardiac enlargement and mediastinal widening (fig. 2.2).

Once the patient's identity has been checked and the film hung properly, it is important to check for any rotation. This can change the shape of the heart and the appearance of the lungs, creating a spurious difference in radiolucency between the two sides. In a properly centered film, the medial ends of the clavicles should be a similar distance from the spinous processes of the thoracic vertebrae.

Remember to look at the periphery of any film as well as its centre. In the case of the chest film, the cervical soft tissues and the upper abdomen should be examined.

If the film appears rather dark, the bones will be well demonstrated, but it will be worth using a bright light to examine the lungs, to avoid missing a small pneumothorax.

The abdominal radiograph

The plain abdominal film is also a commonly requested investigation. Its particular importance in everyday practice is in the demonstration of free intraperitoneal air following bowel perforation or of bowel dilatation and air/fluid levels in intestinal obstruction (fig. 2.3).

It is important to find out about the position of the patient when the film was taken. A patient needs to be erect for at least 10 minutes to permit any free air to accumulate in the typical location below the diaphragm. Lateral "shoot-through" or decubitus films (the latter with the patient lying on one side) can help to establish the presence of a free intraperitoneal air or pneumoperitoneum.

Plain films of the musculoskeletal system

Interpretation of these images is often more straightforward and it is usual, in trauma, to take two views, at right angles to each other. Fractures may be missed on a single view (fig. 2.4).

It is also the case that the soft tissue patterns on a plain film can provide clues to the diagnosis.

Contrast studies of the gastrointestinal tract

High density contrast medium is often used in the investigation of the gastrointestinal (GI) tract. Clinical staff (and medical students) will often be confronted with these studies in clinico-radiological meetings, in the outpatients' clinic and perhaps under examination conditions.

Barium is the commonest contrast medium used and is generally very safe. It is contraindicated in suspected rupture of the GI tract because the presence of barium in the mediastinum or the peritoneum has a very high morbidity rate. In these situations a water-soluble contrast medium, such as gastrografin, is preferred.

Conversely, barium is safer than water-soluble contrast medium in the lungs and in cases where aspiration is suspected, barium should be used. This underlines the importance of providing the radiologist with the relevant clinical information (fig. 2.5).

When interpreting contrast medium studies of the GI tract, such as small bowel follow-through studies and barium enemas, a number of common principles should be applied.

Always try to find out by what route the contrast medium was administered. For instance, a rectal or nasojejunal tube is often visible on the film.

(a)

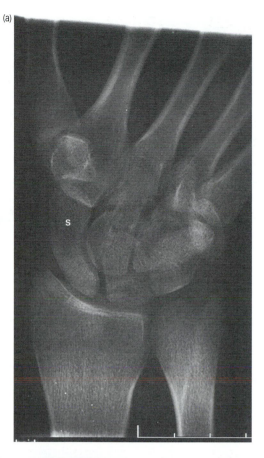

(b)

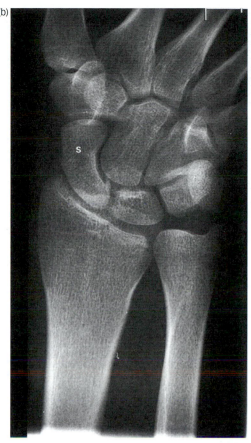

(c)

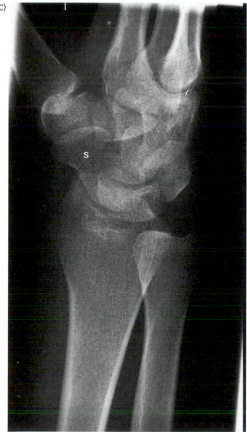

(d)

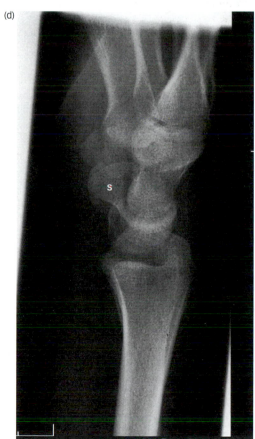

Fig. 2.4. **Multiple views to exclude a fracture of the scaphoid bone. Normal examination.**

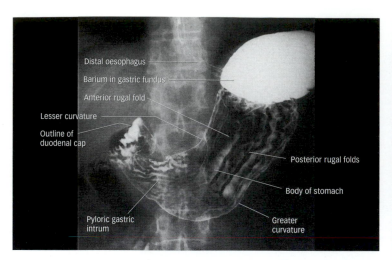

Fig. 2.5. **Supine barium meal examination demonstrating rugal folds. The anterior surface of the stomach can be differentiated from the posterior in the supine position due to pooling of barium around the posterior folds.**

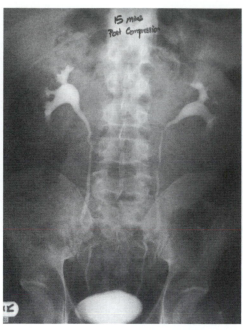

Fig. 2.6. **Intravenous urogram (IVU). 15-minute The renal collecting systems ureters and bladder are opacified with iodinated contrast.**

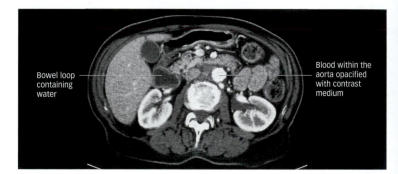

Fig. 2.7. **CT scan upper abdomen, following intravenous contrast medium and water by mouth.**

Establish which part of the bowel has been opacified and how far along the GI tract the contrast medium has travelled. If only the large bowel has been opacified, the study is almost certainly a barium enema.

It may also be useful to establish the position of the patient when the views were taken. fluid levels and bony landmarks are useful for this purpose.

Air is often used as a second contrast medium with barium and these examinations are termed "double-contrast" studies. The distension provided by air insufflation or after swallowing effervescent tablets, as appropriate, results in better mucosal detail.

Bowel preparation is very important in lower GI tract studies as fecal contamination may degrade a barium enema by obscuring a genuine abnormality or by generating artifactual "filling defects." It may help if such defects alter their position between films, confirming their fecal nature.

Similarly, the stomach must be empty of food before a barium meal.

Contrast studies of the kidney and urinary tract

The most common renal contrast medium study performed is the intravenous urogram or "IVU." After a "control" (plain), film has been taken, iodinated contrast medium is injected intravenously and further images are then taken as the contrast medium is excreted through the kidneys. It is important to study the control film carefully to look for calcification, which may subsequently be obscured by contrast medium.

IVU films are taken at different time intervals, which are marked on the film, and an abdominal compression band may be applied to optimize urinary tract opacification (fig. 2.6).

Computed tomography

The principles of computed tomography (CT) have been discussed in the previous chapter. Several points should be remembered in the interpretation of the images.

The images are usually acquired in the axial plane and are viewed as though looking at the patient from the feet up towards the head.

Therefore, the right side of the patient is on the left side of the image, when the images have been acquired with the patient supine.

Oral and intravenous contrast media are often used during a CT scan. Oral contrast medium is usually a water-soluble substance, such as gastrografin. This opacifies the bowel lumen, which becomes hyperdense (white). The bowel can then be differentiated from other soft tissues. Be aware, though, that it is rare for every loop of bowel to be opacified, and unopacified loops may still cause confusion. More recently, water has used as an alternative oral contrast medium. This appears of intermediate density on CT scans, and gives very good delineation of the higher density bowel mucosa adjacent to it (fig. 2.7).

Intravenous contrast medium can be identified on CT scans by the density of the blood within the blood vessels. The aorta is easiest to identify and will appear whiter than the surrounding soft tissues when contrast medium has been used. It is usual for images to be annotated, albeit often rather cryptically with "+C," to inform the radiologist that contrast medium has been administered. Use all the clues available!

The radiodensity of soft tissues will vary depending on the time interval between the administration of the contrast medium and the scan. Scans performed within 20–40 seconds of the injection, termed the arterial phase, will show the aorta very white, but the solid organs

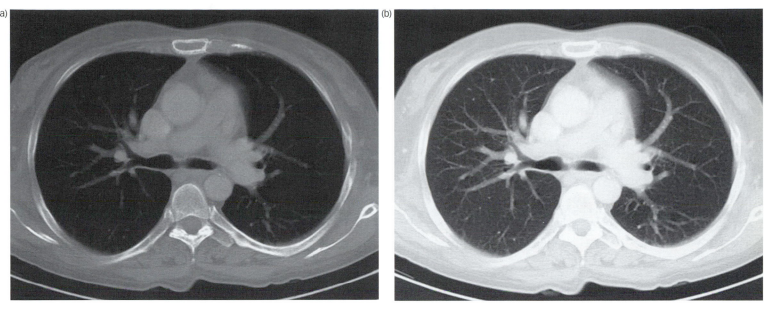

Fig. 2.8. **CT chest. The same image displayed on (a) soft tissue and b) lung windows Mediastinal detail is better shown in (a), pulmonary detail in (b).**

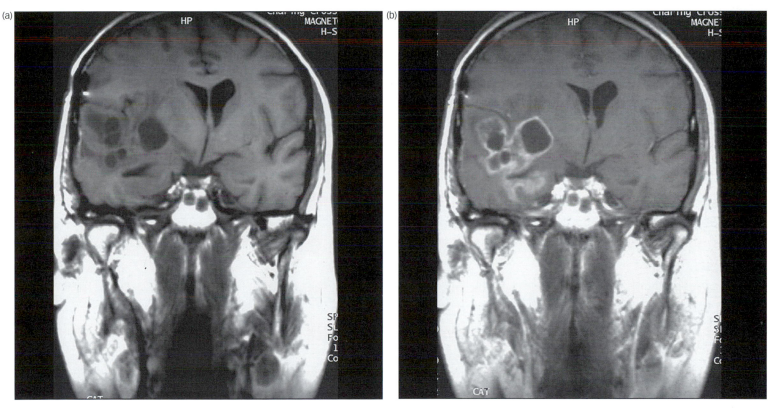

Fig. 2.9. **MRI brain; T1 weighted coronal scans (a) before and (b) after intravenous gadolinium DTPA. Malignant intracerebral tumour. Breakdown of the blood–brain barrier has resulted in gadolinium enhancement of the solid elements of the tumor.**

will not appear to be very different in density from the non-enhanced study. Delayed imaging, at 50–70 seconds, will show the organs to be much brighter. Focal lesions within the liver and spleen are much easier to see on these later images.

As in conventional radiography, calcification can be obscured by the presence of contrast medium, and is best evaluated on a non-enhanced study.

Since it is a digital technique, CT images can be viewed on different "windows." This means that the gray scale of the image is altered so that some tissues are better seen than others (fig. 2.8). The most frequently used windows are for the soft tissues and the lungs. Be sure to look at the appropriate images, so as not to miss important details in the lungs or mediastinum. It is also valuable to view the images on bone windows, to evaluate the presence of focal bone lesions.

CT images are often of varying slice thickness. The slice thickness is written on the images. Thin slices give finer detail but these scans take longer and involve more radiation dose to the patient. Thicker slices can be prone to artifact. High-resolution images of the chest give very fine detail of the lungs.

Magnetic resonance imaging

Magnetic resonance imaging (MRI) is the mainstay of neuroimaging and perhaps also musculoskeletal imaging and is becoming increasingly popular in the evaluation of the hepatobiliary system and pelvis.

The principles of magnetic resonance have been discussed previously. The interpretation of the images can be daunting at first, partly due to the sheer number involved. Images can be acquired in any plane but the commonest are the sagittal, axial and coronal (the orthogonal) planes. It is vital to orientate oneself carefully, by studying the anatomy of the image, before proceeding in the interpretation of the study.

The commonest MR images are T1 or T2 weighted. T2 weighted images show water as white. Most images will show cerebrospinal fluid, which is mainly water, somewhere on the image and this is a useful reference point to decide on the weighting of the scan.

T1 weighted images show fat as very bright, so evaluation of the subcutaneous tissues is helpful in identifying the weighting. There are many other, often complicated, sequences, but a discussion of these is beyond the scope of this introduction.

Gadolinium DTPA is the standard intravenous contrast medium used in MR imaging. It is seen best on T1 weighted images and the principles involved are very similar to those in CT contrast medium enhancement (fig. 2.9).

Other contrast media are used in the evaluation of the hepatobiliary system and of lymph nodes. These agents alter the signal returned from the soft tissues, to increase the conspicuity of focal lesions.

Nuclear medicine imaging

Nuclear medicine images are functional studies and, as such, are interpreted differently. Renal imaging is acquired from the back, so that the right kidney is on the right of the image. Most other images are acquired from the front. The agent used is almost invariably marked on the film and gives important clues to the evaluation of the study. Other helpful clues may be the time of the image acquisition and the use of other agents such as diuretics.

Section 2 | The thorax

Chapter 3 | The chest wall and ribs

JONATHAN D. BERRY
and SUJAL R. DESAI

Introduction

Radiological investigation of the chest is a common occurrence in clinical practice. Thus, a working knowledge of thoracic anatomy, as seen on radiological examinations, is crucial and has an important bearing on management. The present chapter considers the anatomy of the thorax as related to imaging. The appearances of the thoracic structures on plain radiography and computed tomography (which together constitute two of the most frequently requested radiological tests) will be discussed in most detail.

For the purposes of anatomic description, the thorax is bounded by the vertebral column posteriorly, together with the ribs, intercostal muscles, and the sternum antero-laterally. The superior extent of the thorax (lying roughly at the level of the first vertebral body) is the narrowest point and, through the thoracic inlet, the contents of the chest communicate with those of the neck. Inferiorly, the thorax is separated from the abdomen by the diaphragm.

Commonly used techniques for imaging the chest

Imaging of the thorax rightly is regarded as an important component of clinical investigation. For most patients, the plain chest radiograph will be the first (and sometimes only) radiological test that is required. In more complex cases, the clinician will request computed tomography (CT). The technique of magnetic resonance imaging (MRI), which is well established in other spheres of medicine, has relatively few applications for the routine investigation of chest diseases and will not be discussed in any detail in this chapter except where points of anatomical interest can be illustrated.

Chest radiography

The standard projection for imaging of the chest is the postero-anterior (PA) or "frontal" view, in which the patient faces the film plate and the X-ray tube is sited behind the patient. On a frontal projection, because the heart is as close as possible to the X-ray film plate, magnification is minimized (Fig. 3.1). However, in some patients, who are unable to be positioned for the PA view, the antero-posterior projection will become mandatory. Occasionally, when the anatomical localization of lung abnormalities is difficult to discern, a lateral view of the chest will be requested.

Computed tomography (CT)

Computed tomography (CT) is a specialized X-ray technique, which produces cross-sectional (or axial) images of the body. The basic components of a CT machine are an X-ray tube, a series of detectors (sited diametrically opposite the tube), and computer hardware to reconstruct the images. When reviewing CT images, the observer must imagine that the cross-sectional images are being viewed from below; thus, structures on the left of the side of the subject will be on the observer's right.

The main advantage of CT, over plain chest radiography, is that there is no superimposition of anatomical structures. Furthermore, because CT is very sensitive to difference in density of structures and the data are digitized, images may be manipulated to evaluate separately at the pulmonary parenchyma, mediastinal soft tissues, or the ribs and vertebrae (Fig. 3.2).

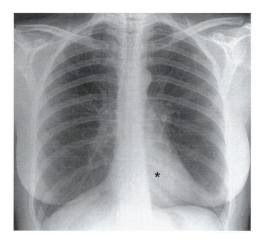

Fig. 3.1. **Standard postero-anterior chest radiograph. The heart (*asterisk*) is of normal size; the ratio of the transverse diameter of the heart to the maximal transverse diameter of the thorax (also called the cardiothoracic ratio) is less than 50%.**

Applied Radiological Anatomy for Medical Students. Paul Butler, Adam Mitchell, and Harold Ellis (eds.) Published by Cambridge University Press. © P. Butler, A. Mitchell, and H. Ellis 2007.

(a)

(b)

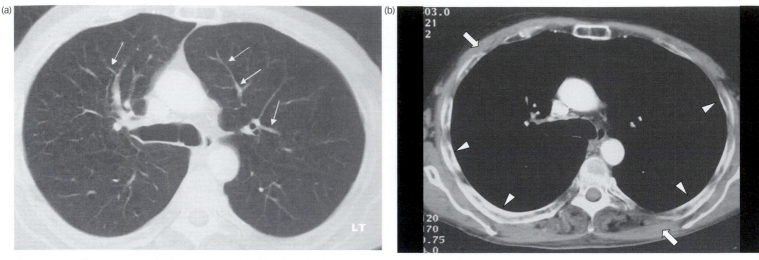

Fig. 3.2. **Two CT images at exactly the same anatomical level manipulated to show (a) the lung parenchyma; the pulmonary vessels are seen as white, branching linear structures (*thin arrows*). (b) Soft-tissue settings showing the midline structures of the mediastinum, ribs (*arrowheads*) and muscles of the chest wall (*thick arrows*) but not the lung parenchyma.**

(a)

(b)

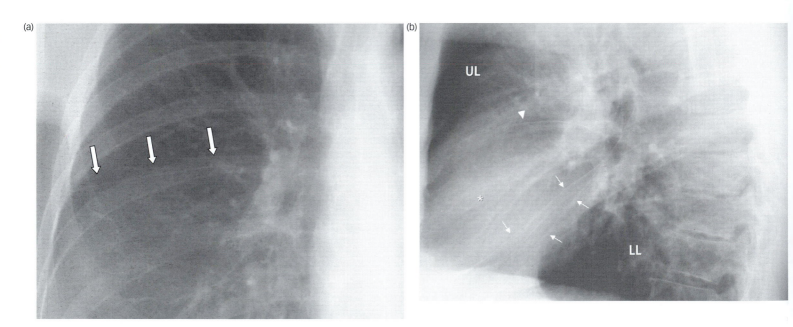

Fig. 3.3. Targeted views of (a) frontal radiograph to show the horizontal (minor) fissure (*arrows*) and (b) lateral projection showing the lower halves of both oblique fissures (*arrows*). The horizontal fissure is also noted on this view (*arrowhead*). The lower lobes (LL) lie behind and below whereas the upper lobes (UL) are above and in front of the oblique fissures. The middle lobe (*asterisk*) is located between the horizontal and relevant oblique fissure.

Anatomy of the chest

The lungs and airways

Each lung occupies, and almost completely fills, its respective hemithorax. On the right, there are three lobes (the upper, middle, and lower) and on the left, two (the upper and lower); incidentally, the lingula generally is considered a part of the left upper lobe. The upper and lower lobes, on each side, are separated from each other by the oblique fissure. On the right, the middle lobe is divided from the upper by the horizontal fissure. By contrast, it should be noted that, on the left, there is no fissural division between the left upper lobe and lingula. On a PA chest radiograph, the oblique fissure is generally not visible. Futhermore, because the upper lobe lies anteriorly, most of the lung that is seen on the frontal view will be the upper lobe.

The horizontal fissure is seen readily on a standard PA radiograph as a thin line crossing from the lateral edge of the hemithorax to the hilum. On a lateral view of the chest, both the oblique fissures may be visualized, running obliquely in a cranio-caudal distribution (Fig. 3.3); the horizontal fissure can also be seen running forward from the oblique fissure Occasionally, accessory fissures will be seen on a chest radiograph.

The lungs are lined by two layers of pleura, which are continuous at the hila. The parietal pleura covers the inner surface of the chest wall whereas the visceral layer is closely applied to the lung surface. A small volume of "normal" pleural fluid is generally present within the pleural cavity to facilitate the smooth movement of one layer over the other during breathing. In the absence of disease, the pleural layers will not be seen on chest radiograph. However, because of the superior contrast resolution, the normal pleura may be visualized on CT images (Fig. 3.4).

The trachea is a vertically orientated tube (measuring approximately 13 cm in length), which commences below the cricoid cartilage and extends to the approximate level of the sternal angle where is bifurcates. In cross-section the outline of the trachea may vary from being oval to a D-shape, depending on the phase of breathing cycle. Anteriorly and laterally, the trachea is bounded by hoops of hyaline cartilage but posteriorly there is a relatively pliable membrane. On a chest radiograph, the trachea is seen as a tubular region of lucency in the midline, as it passes through the thoracic inlet (Fig. 3.5). At the level of the aortic arch, there may be slight (but entirely normal) deviation of the trachea to the right. At the level of the carina, the trachea divides into right and left main bronchi; the former is shorter, wider and more vertically oriented than its counterpart on the left (Fig. 3.6). Each main bronchus gives rise to lobar bronchi, which divide to supply the bronchopulmonary segments in each lobe. Individual bronchopulmonary segments are not readily identified (on chest radiography or CT) but it is worth revising the anatomy because segmental

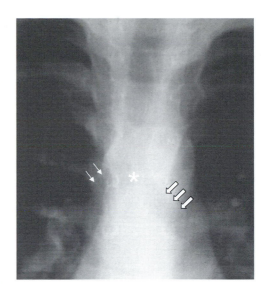

Fig. 3.6. **Targeted and magnified view of the tracheal carina (*asterisk*). The right main bronchus (*thin arrows*) is shorther and more vertically orientated than the left (*thick arrows*).**

airways and arteries can be seen particularly well on CT images and such information may be important to clinicians. On the right, there are ten segments (three in the upper lobe, two in the middle and five in the lower lobe), whereas on the left there are nine (three in upper lobe, two in the lingula and four in the lower lobe (Fig. 3.7).

The mediastinum

For descriptive purposes, the mediastinum has always been thought of in terms of its arbitrary compartments. Thus, the superior mediastinum is considered to lie above a horizontal line drawn from the lower border of the manubrium, the sternal angle or angle of Louis, to the lower border of T4 and below the thoracic inlet (Fig. 3.8). The inferior compartment, lying below this imaginary line (and above the hemidiaphragm) is further subdivided: the anterior mediastinum lies in front of the pericardium and root of the aorta. The middle mediastinum comprises the heart and pericardium together with hilar structures, whereas the posterior mediastinum lies between the posterior aspect of the pericardium and the spine. Whilst the above division is entirely arbitrary, the validity of remembering such a scheme is that the differential diagnosis of mediastinal masses is refined by considering the localization of a mass in a particulary mediastinal compartment. The main contents of the different mediastinal compartments are listed in Table 3.1. Some of the important components of the mediastinum are discussed below:

The esophagus

The esophagus extends from the pharynx (opposite the C6 vertebral body) through the diaphragm (at the level of T10) to the gastroesophageal junction and measures approximately 25 cm in length. In its intrathoracic course the esophagus is a predominantly a left-sided structure, a feature which is readily appreciated on CT images (Fig. 3.9). By contrast, the esophagus is normally not visible on a standard PA radiograph, and radiographic examination requires the patient to drink a radioopaque liquid (i.e., a barium suspension).

The thymus

The thymus is a bilobed structure, which is posititoned in the space between the great vessels (arising from the aorta) and the anterior

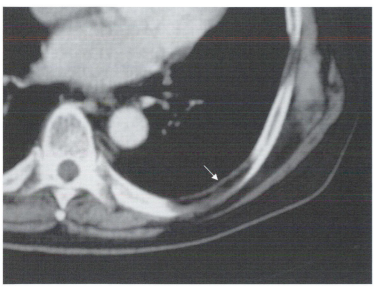

Fig. 3.4. **Targeted view of the left lower zone on CT showing normal thin pleura (*arrow*).**

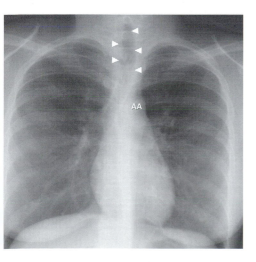

Fig. 3.5. **PA chest showing the characteristic tubular lucency of the trachea (*arrowheads*). The normal and minimal deviation of the trachea to the right is noted at the level of the aortic arch (AA).**

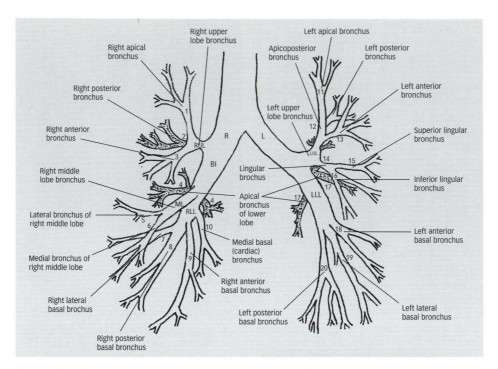

Fig. 3.7. Schematic diagram illustrating the segmental anatomy of the bronchial tree (reproduced with permission from *Applied Radiological Anatomy*, 1st edn, Chapter 6, The chest, p. 129, Fig. 11(f), ed. P. Butler; Cambridge University Press).

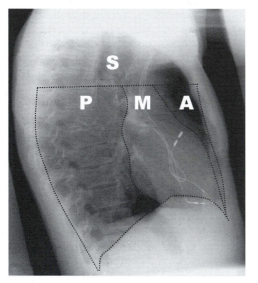

Fig. 3.8. **Lateral radiograph demonstrating the anterior (A), middle (M), posterior (P) and superior (S) mediastinal compartments.**

chest wall. The volume of the thymus normally changes with age: in the newborn, for example, the thymus may occupy the entire volume of the mediastinum anterior to the great vessels (Fig. 3.10). With age, the thymus initially hypertrophies, but after puberty there is progressive atrophy, such that in normal adults, the normal thymus is barely discernible.

The hilum

The hilum can be considered to be the region at which pulmonary vessels and airways enter or exit the lungs. The main components of each hilum are the pulmonary artery, bronchus, veins, and lymph nodes. On a frontal radiograph, the right hilum may be identified as a broad V-shaped structure; the left hilum is often more difficult to identify confidently (Fig. 3.11). A useful landmark for the radiologist,

TABLE 3.1. **American Thoracic Society definitions of regional nodal stations**

X	Supraclavicular nodes
2R	Right upper paratracheal nodes: nodes to the right of the midline of the trachea, between the intersection of the caudal margin of the innominate artery with the trachea and the apex of the lung
2L	Left upper paratracheal nodes: nodes to the left of the midline of the trachea, between the top of the aortic arch and the apex of the lung
4R	Right lower paratracheal nodes: nodes to the right of the midline of the trachea, between the cephalic border of the azygos vein and the intersection of the caudal margin of the brachiocephalic artery with the right side of the trachea
4L	Left lower paratracheal nodes: nodes to the left of the midline of the trachea, between the top of the aortic arch and the level of the carina, medial to the ligamentum arteriosum
5	Aortopulmonary nodes: subaortic and paraaortic nodes, lateral to the ligamentum arteriosum or the aorta or left pulmonary artery, proximal to the first branch of the left pulmonary artery
6	Anterior mediastinal nodes: nodes anterior to the ascending aorta or the innominate artery
7	Subcarinal nodes: nodes arising caudal to the carina of the trachea but not associated with the lower lobe bronchi or arteries within the lung
8	Paraesophageal nodes: nodes dorsal to the posterior wall of the trachea and to the right or left of the midline of the esophagus
9	Right or left pulmonary ligament nodes: nodes within the right or left pulmonary ligament
10R	Right tracheobronchial nodes: nodes to the right of the midline of the trachea, from the level of the cephalic border of the azygos vein to the origin of the right upper lobe bronchus
10L	Left tracheobronchial nodes: nodes to the left of the midline of the trachea, between the carina and the left upper lobe bronchus, medial to the ligamentum arteriosum
11	Intrapulmonary nodes: nodes removed in the right or left lung specimen, plus those distal to the main-stem bronchi or secondary carina

From Glazer et al. (1985).

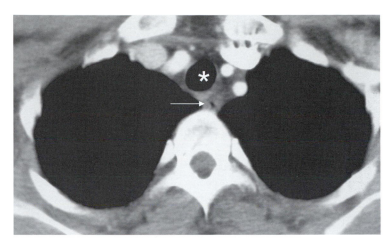

Fig. 3.9. **Axial CT image on soft tissue window settings at the level of the great vessels. The oesophagus (*arrow*) can seen lying just to the left of the midline and posterior to the trachea (*asterisk*).**

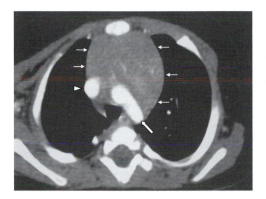

Fig. 3.10. **CT of the normal thymus in an infant. There is a well-defined mass (*thin arrows*) in the superior mediastinum. Note how the mass conforms to the outline of some the major vessels (the aorta [*thick arrow*] and superior vena cava (*arrowhead*)) in the mediastinum, and does not displace them.**

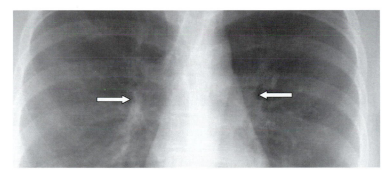

Fig. 3.11. **Targeted and magnified view from PA chest radiograph clearly shows the hilar vessels. The right and left hilar points (where the upper lober veins apparently "cross" the lower lobe artery) are indicated (*arrows*).**

on the PA radiograph, is the so-called "hilar point" which, whilst not being a true anatomical structure, is the apparent region where the upper lobe pulmonary veins meet the lower pulmonary artery. In normal subjects, the hilar point is sited roughly between the apex and the base of the hemithorax: in some patients, significant elevation or depression of the hilar point will be the only clue to the presence of volume loss in the lungs.

The heart

In the embryo, the heart is one of the earliest organs to develop, following fusion of two parallel tubular structures known as the

primitive aortae; with subsequent septation and coiling, the characteristic asymmetric configuration of the adult heart is attained. The pericardium, which like the pleura is a two-layered membrane, encases the heart; the inner (or visceral) pericardium is applied directly to the myocardium except for a region that reflects around the pulmonary veins. The outer (parietal) pericardium is continuous with the adventitial fibrous covering of the great vessels. Inferiorly, the parietal pericardium blends with the central tendon of the diaphragm. As with the pleura, the potential space between the visceral and parietal pericardium (the pericardial sac) is not normally visible on plain radiographs. Again, because of the superior contrast resolution of CT, the normal pericardial lining may be identified on axial images.

In normal subjects there are four cardiac chambers (the paired atria and ventricles). Deoxygenated blood is normally delivered to the right atrium via the superior vena cava (from the upper limbs, thorax, via the azygos sytem, and the head and neck), the inferior vena cava (from the lower limbs and abdomen), and the coronary sinus (from the myocardium). The right atrium is separated from its counterpart on the left by the inter-atrial septum which, with the changes in pressure that occur at or soon after birth, normally seals; a depression in the interatrial septum marks the site of the foramen ovale in the fetal heart. The right atrium is a "border-forming" structure on a PA radiograph that is immediately adjacent to the medial segment of the right middle lobe, a feature that is readily appreciated on CT images (Fig. 3.12). The right ventricle communicates with the atrium via the tricuspid valve. Deoxygenated blood leaves the right ventricle through the pulmonary valve and enters the pulmonary arterial tree. Because the right ventricle is an anterior chamber, it does not form a border on the standard PA radiograph but the outline of the chamber is visible on a lateral radiograph. The left atrium is a smooth-walled chamber and is posteriorly positioned. Oxygenated blood enters the atrium from the paired pulmonary veins on each side and exits via the mitral valve to the left ventricle from where blood is delivered into the systemic circulation. As on the right, there is a left atrial appendage (sometimes referred to as the auricular appendage), which may be the only part of the normal atrium that is seen on the frontal radiograph; conversely, the wall of the left atrium is easily identified on a lateral radiograph.

The left ventricle is the most muscular cardiac chamber and is a roughly cone-shaped structure whose axis is oriented along the left anterior oblique plane. On a frontal chest radiograph, the left ventricle accounts for most of the left heart border. It is worth mentioning at this point that the widest transverse diameter of the heart (extending from the right (formed by the right atrium) to the left margin) is an important measurement on the frontal radiograph: as a general rule, the transverse diameter should be less than half the maximal diameter of the chest (this measurement is called the cardiothoracic ratio).

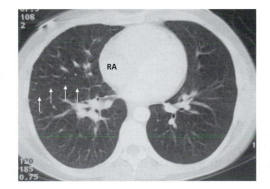

Fig. 3.12. **Axial CT image on lung parenchymal window settings showing the relationship of the middle lobe (lying anterior to the horizontal fissure [arrows]), particularly its medial segment and the right atrium (RA).**

(a)

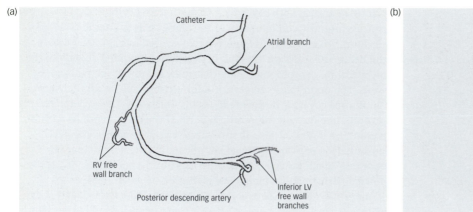

(b)

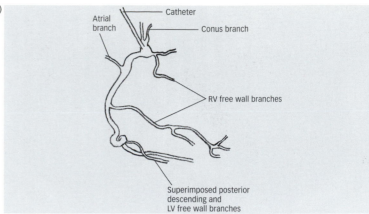

Fig. 3.13 (a), (b). **Coronary angiogram demonstrating the left and right coronary arteries (reproduced with permission from *Applied Radiological Anatomy*, 1st edn, Chapter 7, The heart and great vessels, p. 165, Figs. 24 and 25; ed. P. Butler, Cambridge University Press).**

Oxygenated blood normally enters the ventricle from the left atrium via the mitral valve and is pumped into the systemic circulation through the aortic valve. Just above the aortic valve there are three focal dilatations, called the sinuses of Valsalva. The right coronary artery originates from the anterior sinus, whilst the left posterior sinus gives rise to the left coronary artery; the coronary circulation is described as either right (the most common arrangement) or left dominant depending on which vessel supplies the posterior diaphragmatic region of the interventricular septum and diaphragmatic surface of the left ventricle. The right coronary artery usually runs forward between the pulmonary trunk and right auricle. As it descends in the atrioventricular groove, branches arise to supply the right atrium and ventricle. At the inferior border of the heart, it continues and ultimately unites with the left coronary artery. The larger left coronary artery descends between the pulmonary trunk and left auricle, and runs in the left atrioventricular groove for about 1 cm before dividing into the left anterior descending (interventricular) artery and the circumflex arteries. In around one-third of normal subjects, the left coronary artery will trifurcate and in such cases there is a "ramus medianus" or "intermediate" artery between the left anterior descending and circumflex arteries supplying the anterior left ventricular wall. The venous drainage of the heart is via the coronary sinus (which enters the right atrium) and receives four main tributaries: the great cardiac vein, middle cardiac vein, small cardiac vein, and left posterior ventricular vein. A smaller proportion of the venous drainage is directly into the right atrium via the anterior cardiac veins that enter the anterior surface of the right atrium. As might be imagined, the normal cardiac circulation is not seen on standard radiographic examinations. However, the injection of intravenous contrast via a coronary artery catheter (inserted retrogradely via the femoral artery) will render the vessels visible (Fig. 3.13). An alternative approach (which has only become possible since the advent of "fast" CT scanning machines) is for the cardiac circulation to be imaged following a peripheral injection of contrast. More recently, there has been considerable interest in the imaging of the heart and its circulation using magnetic resonance imaging.

The aorta

The intrathoracic aorta can conveniently be considered in four parts: the root, the ascending aorta, the arch, and the descending aorta. The root comprising the initial few centimeters, is invested by

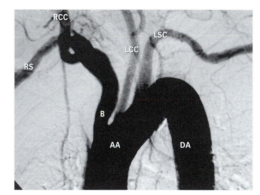

Fig. 3.14. **Digital subtraction angiogram showing the ascending (AA) and descending (DA) aorta. Note that the brachiocephalic artery (B) bifurcates into the right subclavian (RS) and right common carotid (RCC) arteries; the left common carotid (LCC) and left subclavian (LSC) also arise from the aortic arch.**

pericardium and includes three focal dilatations, the sinuses of Valsalva (described above) above the aortic valve leaflets. The ascending aorta continues upward and to the right for approximately 5 cm to the level of the sternal angle. The arch lies inferior to the manubrium sterni and is directed upward, inferiorly, and to the left. The arch initally lies anterior to the trachea and esophagus, but then extends to the bifurcation of the pulmonary trunk. The three important branches of the aortic arch are the brachiocephalic artery, the left common carotid artery, and the left subclavian artery, all of which are readily visible on angiographic studies and CT (Fig. 3.14). Variations to this normal pattern of branching occur in approximately one-third of subjects; the most common variant is that in which the left common carotid arises from the brachiocephalic artery.

By convention, the descending aorta begins at the point of attachment of the ligamentum arteriosum to the left pulmonary artery (roughly at the level of T4). The descending aorta passes downward in the posterior mediastinum on the left to the level of T12, where it passes through the diaphragm and into the abdomen. Within the thorax, the descending aorta gives rise to the intercostal, subcostal arteries, bronchial, esophageal, spinal, and superior phrenic arteries.

Pulmonary arteries

At its origin from the right ventricle, the pulmonary conus or trunk is invested by a pericardial reflection. The main divisions of trunk are the left and right pulmonary arteries. The right pulmonary artery passes in front of the right main bronchus and behind the ascending aorta. Anteriorly, the right superior pulmonary vein crosses the right

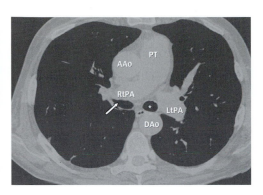

Fig. 3.15. **CT image just below the level of the tracheal carina. The right main pulmonary artery (RtPA) passes in front of the right main bronchus (*arrow*). The left pulmonary artery arches over the left main bronchus (*asterisk*). AAo = ascending aorta; PT = pulmonary trunk; LtPA = left basal pulmonary artery.**

main artery (Fig. 3.15). At the hilum, the artery divides into the upper and lower divisions, from which the lobar and segmental branches orginate; It is important to remember that arterial branching (unlike the pulmonary veins) closely follows the branching of the airways. The left main pulmonary artery passes posteriorly from the pulmonary trunk and then arches over the left main bronchus. As with the coronary arteries, the pulmonary circulation is visualized optimally after the injection of intravenous contrast, as in conventional pulmonary angiography (a technique seldom performed in modern radiology departments) or on CT images. The venous drainage of the lungs is via the left and right pulmonary veins, two on each side, which enter the left atrium beneath the level of the pulmonary arteries. Occasionally, the veins can be seen to unite prior to their entry into the left atrium.

It should be remembered that, in addition to the main pulmonary arterial supply, there is a bronchial circulation originating from the systemic circulation. The most common arrangement is of a single right bronchial artery (usually arising from the third posterior intercostal) and two left bronchial arteries (originating from the descending thoracic aorta). However, there is considerable normal variation. There are two groups of bronchial veins: the deep veins taking blood from the lung parenchyma and draining into the pulmonary veins. The superficial bronchial veins receive blood from the extrapulmonary bronchi, visceral pleura, and hilar lymph nodes, both draining into the pulmonary veins. The bronchial vessels, although small, are of great clinical importance. They maintain perfusion of the lung after a pulmonary embolism so that, if the patient recovers, the affected lung returns to normal.

The thoracic duct

The thoracic duct is the main channel by which lymph is returned to the circulation. The thoracic duct begins within the abdomen as a dilated sac known as the cistrna chyla and ascends through the diaphragm on the right of the aorta. At the level of the sixth thoracic vertebral body, the thoracic duct crosses to the left of the spine and passes upwards to arch over the subclavian artery. The duct drains lymph into a large central vein, which is close to the union of the left internal jugular and subclavian veins. The diameter of the thoracic duct may vary between 2 and 8 mm and, although usually single, multiple channels may exist. In normal subjects, the thoracic duct is collapsed and, as such, cannot be visualized on imaging studies. A variation on the normal is for a right-sided lymphatic duct, which drains lymph from the right side of the thorax, the right upper limb, and right head and neck into the right brachiocephalic vein.

The thoracic cage

Ribs, sternum and vertebrae

The thorax is roughly cylindrical in shape and shielded by the ribs, thoracic vertebrae, and the sternum. All 12 pairs of ribs are attached posteriorly to their respective vertebral bodies. In addition, the upper seven pairs attach anteriorly to the sternum via individual costal cartilages. The eighth, ninth and tenth ribs effectively are attached to each other and also the seventh rib by means of a "common" costal cartilage. With age, the costal cartilages may calcify and are then readily visible on a frontal radiograph. The two lowermost ribs (the 11th and 12th) are described as "floating" since they have no anterior attachment. An interesting variation to the normal arrangement (occuring in around 6% of the population) is the so-called "cervical" rib, which articulates with a cervical, instead of a throracic vertebral body (Fig. 3.16). Cervical ribs may be uni- or bilateral. Occasionally, there will simply be a fibrous band but, when calcified, the appearance of a "true rib" will be seen. Some cervical ribs are symptomatic because of the potential for compression of the subclavian artery and first thoracic nerve root.

The sternum can be considered to comprise three components: the manubrium sterni, the body of the sternum, and the xiphoid process (or xiphisternum). The manubrium is the uppermost and widest portion, which articulates laterally with the clavicles and also the first and upper part of the second costal cartilages; inferiorly, the manubrium articulates with the body of the sternum. On a conventional frontal chest radiograph, the bulk of the manubrium is generally not visible. However, the articulation of the manubrium with the clavicles (the manubrio-clavicular joint) can be seen. By contrast, on a lateral radiograph the manubrium can be clearly identified. The body of the sternum is a roughly rectangular structure which has a notched lateral margin, where it articulates with the costal cartilages of the third to seventh ribs. The xiphoid is the most inferior portion of the sternum and prinicipally consists of hyaline cartilage that may become ossified in later life.

The thoracic vertebrae provide structural support to the thorax in both the axial (vertical) and, through the attachment with ribs and muscles, the coronal and sagittal planes. Whilst individual vertebrae are rigid, their articulations mean there is considerable potential mobility in terms of flexion, extension, and rotational movements over the length of the twelve vertebrae. There is a progressive increase in the height of thoracic vertebrae bodies from T1 to T12 and these vertebrae can be distinguished by the presence of lateral facets, which articulate with the heads of the ribs. Facet joints for articulation with the tubercles of the ribs are also present on the transverse processes of T1 to T10. Furthermore, when viewed in the sagittal plane, each

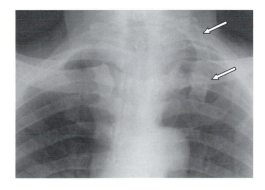

Fig. 3.16. **Targeted view from a PA chest radiograph demonstrating a unilateral left sided calcified cervical rib (*arrows*).**

vertebrae can be seen to possess a long spinous process; with the exception of T1 (whose spinous process is almost horizontal), the spinous processes all point downward.

Initial analysis of the thoracic vertebrae is still best done with a suitably penetrated plane film. However, in the presence of complex trauma or where the contents of the spinal canal need to be visualized, CT and MRI are being employed increasingly.

Muscles of the chest wall

There is a complex arrangement of muscles around the chest which, in addition to the vital act of breating, help to maintain stability. Outermost and anteriorly are the pectoralis (major and minor) muscles; serratus anterior is situated laterally, and posterolaterally are the muscles of the shoulder girdle. Posteriorly and adjacent to the vertebrae are erector spinae and trapezius. These muscle groups are readily depicted on axial (CT and MRI) images (Fig. 3.17). The deeper muscles of the chest include the intercostal muscles (external, internal, and innermost), which are situated between the ribs. Elsewhere, the subcostal muscles span several ribs and further muscles attach the ribs to the sternum and vertebrae. All these muscles may be visualized accurately with MR.

Each intercostal space is supplied by a single large posterior intercostal artery and paired anterior intercostal arteries. Incidentally, each posterior intercostal artery also gives off a spinal branch, which supplies the vertebrae and spinal cord. The venous drainage is via the posterior intercostal veins running backward to drain into the azygos (or hemi-azygos) and the anterior intercostal veins into the internal thoracic and musculophrenic veins.

Nerve supply of the chest wall

The innervation of the chest wall is via 12 paired thoracic nerves. The 11 pairs of intercostal nerves run between the ribs while the twelfth pair (the subcostal nerves) runs below the twelfth rib in the anterior abdominal wall. The intercostal nerves are the anterior rami of the first 11 thoracic spinal nerves, which enter the intercostal space between the parietal pleura and posterior intercostal membrane to run in the subcostal groove of the corresponding ribs and below the intercostal artery and vein. It is for this reason that, whenever possible, needle aspiration or pleural drainage should be performed by entering the pleural space immediately *above*.

In addition to the peripheral nervous system, the sympathetic chain is also found within the thorax. There are either 11 or 12 sympathetic

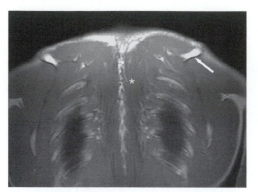

Fig. 3.17. **Coronal magnetic resonance image of the posterior aspect of the thorax at the level of the acromion process of the scapula (*arrow*) showing the erector spinae muscles (*asterisk*).**

ganglia within the thorax. The first ganglia is frequently fused with the inferior cervical ganglia to form the cervicothoracic or "stellate" ganglia. The remaining ganglia are simply numbered so that they correspond to the adjacent segmental structures. A number of plexi are formed through the fusion of different ganglia, for example, the cardiac plexus and aortic plexus.

The diaphragm

The diaphragm is the domed structure, which serves to separate the contents of the thorax from those of the abdomen and plays a vital role in breathing. The components of the diaphragm are a peripheral muscular portion and a central tendon. The diaphragm is fixed to the chest wall at three main points: the vertebral attachment (via the crura which extend down to the level of the lumbar vertebrae), the costal component (comprising slips of muscle attached to the the deep part of the six lowermost ribs), and finally the sternal component (consisting of slips of muscle arising from the posterior aspect of the xiphoid process). At three points, roughly in the midline, the central tendon transmits (and is pierced) by the esophagus, descending aorta, and inferior vena cava.

The normal diapragm is easily visualized on both frontal and lateral radiographs as a smooth but curved structure. Laterally, on the frontal radiograph, the diaphragm appears to make contact with the chest wall. At the apparent point of contact (called the costophrenic recess) the angle subtended to the chest wall is acute and well defined. This is of practical value since even small collections of fluid (pleural effusions) will lead to a blunting of the costophrenic recess.

Section 2 | The thorax

Chapter 4 | The breast

STELLA COMITIS

Breast cancer is the commonest malignancy in women in Europe and the United States. In recent years, physicians and the media have encouraged women to practice self-examination, to have regular evaluation by a medical practitioner, and to participate in breast screening programs. This has resulted in the general population developing a heightened awareness of breast cancer and in turn presenting to the general practitioner with a variety of breast complaints. In order to evaluate properly such symptoms, there must be an understanding of the normal breast. This chapter serves to describe normal breast anatomy and the role of imaging techniques used to evaluate the breast.

Embryology

During the fourth gestational week, paired ectodermal thickenings called mammary ridges (milk lines) develop along the ventral surface of the embryo from the base of the forelimb buds to the hindlimb buds. In the human, only the mammary ridges at the fourth intercostal space will proliferate and form the primary mammary bud, which will branch further into the secondary buds, develop lumina and coalesce to form lactiferous ducts. By term, there are 15–20 lobes of glandular tissue, each with a lactiferous duct. The lactiferous ducts open onto the areola, which develops from the ectodermal layer. The supporting fibrous connective tissue, Cooper's ligaments, and fat in the breast develop from surrounding mesoderm.

At birth, the mammary glands are identical in males and females and remain quiescent until puberty, when ductal growth occurs in females under the influence of estrogens, growth hormones and prolactin. When pregnancy occurs, the glands complete their differentiation by eventually forming secretory alveoli. After the menopause, decreased hormone levels lead to a senescent phase with involution of the glandular component and replacement with connective tissue and fat.

Congenital breast malformations fall into two categories: the presence of supernumerary tissue, or the underdevelopment of breast tissue. If the milk line fails to involute, it results in supernumerary breast tissue. The commonest form, found in 2–5% of the population, is polythelia, which is the presence of two or more nipples along the chest wall in the plane of the embryonic milk line. The absence or underdevelopment of breast tissue is less common. The severity ranges from amastia, the complete absence of glandular tissue, nipple and areola, to hypoplasia, the presence of rudimentary breasts.

Breast anatomy

The adult breast lies on the anterior chest wall between the second rib above and the sixth rib inferiorly, and from the sternal edge medially to the mid-axillary line laterally. Breast tissue also projects into the axilla as the axillary tail of Spence. The breasts lie on the pectoral fascia, covering the pectoralis major and minor muscles medially and serratus anterior and external oblique muscles laterally. The breasts are contained within a fascial sac, which forms when the superficial pectoral fascia splits into anterior (superficial) and posterior (deep) layers. The suspensory Cooper's ligaments are projections of the superficial fascia that run through the breast tissue and connect to subcutaneous tissues and skin.

The nipple is found centrally on each breast and has abundant sensory nerve endings. The lactiferous ducts each open separately on the nipple. Surrounding the nipple is the areola, which is pigmented and measures 15–60 mm. Near the periphery of the areola are elevations (tubercles of Morgagni) formed by the openings of modified sebaceous glands, whose secretion protect the nipple during breastfeeding.

The human breast contains 15–20 lobes. Each of these lobes has a major duct, which connects to, and opens on, the nipple. Each lobe consists of numerous lobules, which in turn are made of numerous *acini* (or ductules). This forms the basis of the terminal ductal lobular unit (TDLU), which is a histological descriptive term. The TDLU is an important structure, as it is postulated that most cancers arise in the terminal duct, either inside or just proximal to the lobule. The ducts are named according to their position along the branching structure. The acini drain into the *intralobular* ducts which drain into the *extralobular* ducts and eventually into the *main duct*, which opens on the nipple. The acini and ducts structures form the glandular breast parenchyma, which is surrounded by fatty tissue and fibrous connective tissue, which forms the stroma.

The glandular breast parenchyma predominates in the anterior third and upper quadrant of the breast. Between the glandular

Applied Radiological Anatomy for Medical Students. Paul Butler, Adam Mitchell, and Harold Ellis (eds.) Published by Cambridge University Press. © P. Butler, A. Mitchell, and H. Ellis 2007.

parenchyma and the pectoral muscle, there is predominantly fatty tissue named the retroglandular tissue.

The relative amounts of glandular breast tissue and stroma alter over the normal lifespan. Younger women have more glandular breast tissue and, with increasing age, this is replaced with fibrofatty tissue, particularly after the menopause. Women who take hormone replacement therapy preserve the glandular breast tissue for a longer period. With pregnancy, the number of acini is increased and this persists in the lactation period. After pregnancy, the acini decrease in number and the breast will be less dense than prior to pregnancy. There is, however, great variation in the composition of breast tissue with some women having fatty breasts throughout their lives and others with extremely dense glandular and fibrous tissue.

Arterial supply

The arterial supply of the breast is derived from branches of the internal thoracic artery, lateral thoracic artery, and posterior intercostal arteries. Venous drainage is primarily into the axillary vein but also into the internal thoracic vein, subclavian vein, and azygos vein.

Nerve supply

Innervation of the breasts is primarily via the anterior and lateral cutaneous branches of the upper six thoracic intercostal nerves.

Lymphatics

Understanding the lymphatic drainage of the breast is vital because of its importance in the spread of malignant disease. The majority (97%) of the lymph from the breast drains to axillary nodes, and approximately 3% drains to the internal thoracic nodes. For surgical purposes, to plan the removal of pathological nodes, the axilla is divided into three arbitrary levels. Level I nodes (low axilla) lie lateral to the lateral border of the pectoralis minor muscle, level II nodes (mid axilla) lie behind the muscle, and the level III nodes (apical axilla) are located medial to the medial border of the pectoralis minor muscle.

The concept of a *sentinel node*, which is defined as the first node that drains a cancer, was first described in relation to melanoma and subsequently adapted to breast tumors. A blue dye (or more recently in combination with a radiolabeled colloid), is injected into the tumor and the identification of this dye in the sentinel node will predict the status of the remaining nodes (95% accuracy).

Normal axillary lymph nodes can be demonstrated on both mammography and ultrasound. On mammography, nodes are oval structures with a lucent centre due to the fatty hilum and should measure less than 2 cm. On ultrasound, normal nodes are oval with a hypoechoic rim and a bright center (Figs. 4.1, 4.2). Arterial and venous supply is seen entering and leaving from the hilum, which can be notched with the result that the lymph node will have a bean-shape.

Imaging

Mammography allows excellent characterization of breast tissue. Special mammography units use low dose radiation to image the breast tissue. Mammography is most suitable for women over the age of 40, as at a younger age the glandular tissue is very dense and differentiation of the tissues is difficult. Mammography can be performed with the patient seated or standing. To maximize the tissue imaged, the breast needs to be pulled away from the chest wall and compressed. Compression creates a uniform thickness through which the X-ray beam penetrates so that a uniform exposure can be obtained. Compression also reduces motion artifact by holding the breast still and by separating overlapping structures.

Two views of each breast are obtained in the first instance: a medio-lateral-oblique (MLO) view and a cranio-caudal (CC) view. The MLO view allows the breast to be viewed in profile, ideally from high in the axilla to the inframammary fold (Fig. 4.3). In the CC projection the breast is viewed as if looking from above the breast downwards. In an adequate CC projection, the nipple is seen in profile and the retroglandular fat should be visible. Generally, more tissue can be projected on

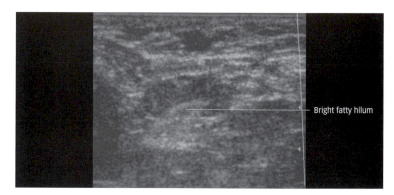

Fig. 4.2. **Ultrasound of the axillary tail demonstrating a normal axillary lymph node with central fatty hilum.**

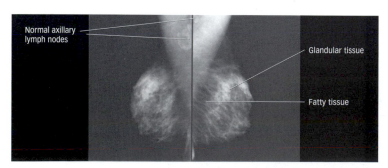

Fig. 4.1. **Mammogram in the mediolateral oblique (MLO) projection, demonstrates normal sized axillary lymph nodes with notched hilum. Note the normal calcified vessels bilaterally.**

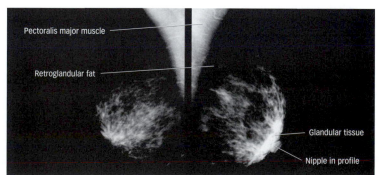

Fig. 4.3. **Mammogram in the mediolateral oblique (MLO) projection. The pectoralis major muscle projects to the level of the nipple and the retroareolar fat is well seen. The nipple is visualized in profile.**

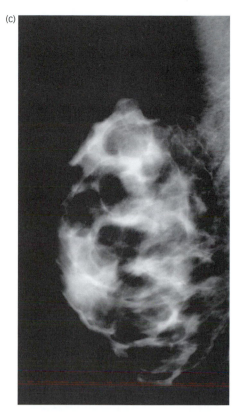
(c)

the MLO projection than on the CC projection because of the slope and curve of the chest wall. The pectoralis major muscle is visualized in only 30–40% of women on a normal CC view (Fig. 4.4).

Normal mammographic patterns

Patterns of normal breast parenchyma vary greatly (Fig. 4.5). The most widely accepted classification of breast patterns is that of Wolfe, which consists of four groups.

Pattern type	Description
N1	Predominantly fatty parenchyma
P1	15–25% nodular densities
P2	>35% nodular densities
DY pattern	Extreme nodularity and density

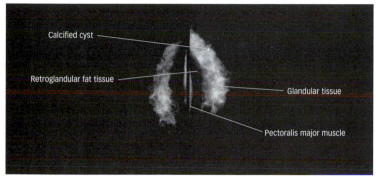

Fig. 4.4. **Mammogram in the cranio-caudal (CC) projection. The retroglandular tissue is seen but the pectoral muscle is only visible in 30–40% of CC projection mammograms.**

(a)
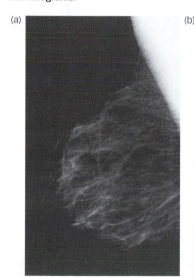

(b)
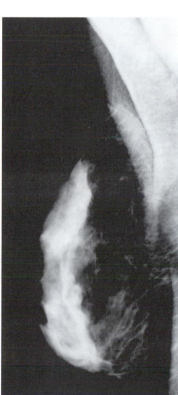

(d)
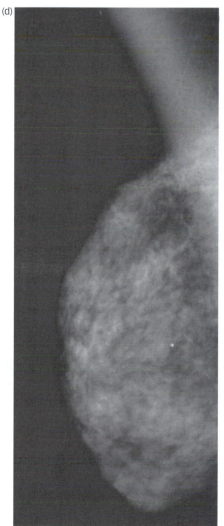

Fig. 4.5. **Wolfe classification of breast parenchymal patterns (a) N1 predominantly fatty tissue (b) P1 is less than 25% nodular tissue (c) P2 is greater than 25% nodular tissue (d) DY pattern is uniformly extremely dense breast tissue.**

Viewing a mammogram

As with all imaging, abnormalities on mammogram are seen as a disruption in the normal anatomical pattern. Mammograms should be viewed back-to-back as mirror images of each other. The breast parenchyma should be symmetrical. Any areas of asymmetry, differing density between the breasts or architectural distortion, should be viewed with suspicion. A magnifying glass should be used to assess areas of microcalcification.

Ultrasound

Since the 1980s, high resolution probes perform "real-time" examination of breast tissue. Breast ultrasound is now seen as the most important adjunct to assessing breast tissue. It is, however, not used alone for routine screening for breast disease. The advantages of ultrasound in imaging the breast include reproducible size evaluation of lesions, differentiation of solid from cystic structures and evaluation and biopsy of abnormalities close to the chest wall and in the periphery of the breast.

The following tissue layers can be differentiated with ultrasound: skin and nipple, subcutaneous fat, glandular tissue and surrounding fibrous tissue, fat lobules, breast ducts, pectoralis major muscle, ribs and intercostal muscle layer. Deep to the ribs, the pleura is identified as a thin, very bright, echogenic layer (Figs. 4.6, 4.7, 4.8). Lymph nodes in the breast and axilla are identifiable as oval structures with low density periphery, a notched hilum, and an echogenic centre.

Magnetic resonance imaging (Fig. 4.9)

Although mammography has revolutionized imaging of the breasts, there are still a number of instances where suboptimal imaging is obtained with mammography. In some breasts, X-rays are severely attenuated, which results in poor penetration and suboptimal visualization of masses. These problems are seen in women with mammographically dense breasts, in the presence of breast prostheses, and in scar tissue.

Magnetic resonance imaging is therefore most useful to assess the integrity of breast implants and normal tissue around the implants, to assess postoperative breast tissue as it allows differentiation of tumour recurrence from scar tissue, and to look for multifocal disease in dense breasts. While MRI is highly sensitive for detection of focal lesions, its specificity for lesion characterization is not as high, and so it should not be used as a solitary imaging modality, but rather as an adjunct to mammography and ultrasound.

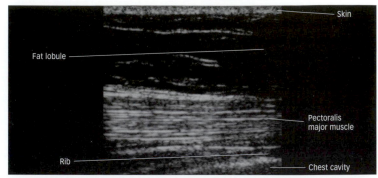

Fig. 4.6. **Ultrasound transverse image demonstrating normal breast parenchyma with lobules of fat interspersed with bright bands of fibrous septa.**

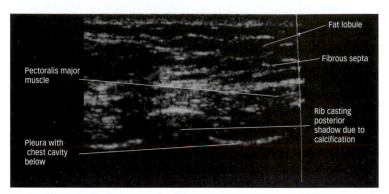

Fig. 4.7. **Ultrasound axial image of axillary tail demonstrates normal breast tissue and the underlying chest wall structures.**

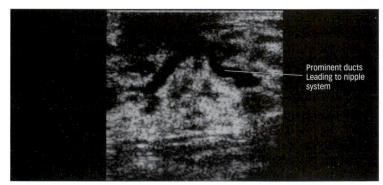

Fig. 4.8. **Ultrasound of the retroareolar region demonstrating prominent breast ducts joining to form a single duct which opens on the nipple.**

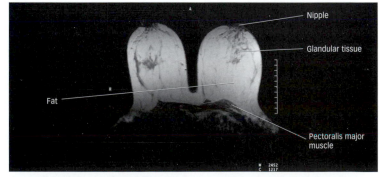

Fig. 4.9. **Axial MRI of the breast tissue demonstrates predominantly fatty breast parenchyma with a little residual glandular tissue in the retroareolar regions.**

Further reading

1 Friederich, M. and Sickles, E. A. (2000). *Radiological Diagnosis of Breast Diseases*. Berlin:Springer Verlag.

2 Kopans, D. B. (1998). *Breast Imaging*. 2nd edn. Philadelphia: Lippincott-Raven.

3 Gray, H. (1999). *Gray's Anatomy*. Courage Books.

4 Husband, J. E. S. and Reznek, R. H. (1998). *Imaging in Oncology*. Oxford: Isis Medical Media.

5 Harris, J. R., Lippman, M. E., Morrow, M., and Osborne, C. K. (2000). *Diseases of the Breast*. 2nd edn. Philadelphia: Lippincott, Williams & Wilkins.

6 Jackson, V. P., Hendrick, R. E., Feig, S. A., and Kopans, D. B. (1993). Imaging of the radiographically dense breast. *Radiology*, **188**, 297–301.

7 Wolfe, J. N. (1976). Breast parenchymal patterns and their changes with age. *Radiology*, **121**, 545–552.

8 Tanis, P. J., Nieweg, O. E., Valdes, Olmos, R. A., Kroon, B. B. (2001). Anatomy and physiology of lymphatic drainage of the breast from the perspective of sentinel node biopsy, *J. Am. Coll. Surg.* **193**(4), 462–465.

9 Tabar, L. and Dean, P. B. (2001). *Teaching Atlas of Mammography*. Thième Medical Publishers.

Section 3 | The abdomen and pelvis

Chapter 5 | The abdomen

DOMINIC BLUNT

The anterior abdominal wall comprises a number of layers. From superficial to deep these are: the skin and superficial fascia layers, subcutaneous fat, muscles and their aponeuroses, extraperitoneal fat, and the peritoneum itself. These layers extend from the xiphoid, lower costal cartilages and ribs to the bones of the pelvic brim inferiorly. The lower ribs and chest wall overlie many structures in the upper abdominal cavity.

The superficial fascia is subdivided into layers and contains predominantly fat, with lymphatics, nerves, and vessels. The fat within it is the most conspicuous component on imaging and the thin fascial layers are continuous with layers of superficial fascia over the thighs and external genitalia inferiorly, and the chest wall superiorly.

The muscles comprise three sheet-like layers (the external oblique, the internal oblique and the transversalis muscles). These become thin aponeuroses medially. Medially are the paired band-like rectus abdominis muscles. Fat and connective tissue can be seen between these layers on imaging (Fig. 5.1).

The superficial muscle layer is the external oblique and its aponeurosis. This originates from the outer aspects of the lower ribs and the muscular slips unite to run inferomedially, continuing as an aponeurosis inserting in the midline into the linea alba (a tough band of connective tissue) where it joins the aponeuroses of the other two sheet-like muscles. Inferiorly, it inserts into the anterior half of the iliac crest and the pubic tubercle, the inferior part of the aponeurosis forming the inguinal ligament, stretching from the anterior superior iliac spine to the pubic tubercle.

The internal oblique originates from the inguinal ligament, the iliac crest, and thoracolumbar fascia. It runs in a broad fan superomedially and its aponeurosis inserts into the lower ribs, the linea alba, and pubis.

The third layer is the transversus abdominis, which runs transversely from the internal aspect of the lower ribs, the thoracolumbar fascia, the iliac crest, and inguinal ligament. Its aponeurosis inserts into the linea alba and inferiorly into the pubic tubercle.

Medially, the common aponeurosis of these three muscles forms the rectus sheath, which in the upper abdomen forms layers anterior and posterior to the rectus muscle; in the lower abdomen the sheath runs only anterior to it.

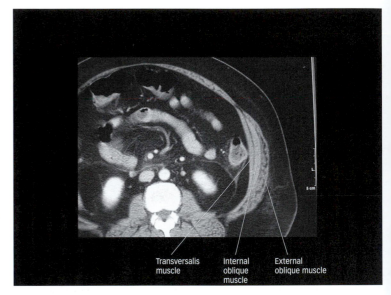

Fig. 5.1. **Axial CT image at the level of the lower pole of the kidneys. Note the rectus abdominis muscles joined in the midline, and laterally the three layers (external oblique, internal oblique and thin transversalis), whose fascia can be seen passing deep to the rectus muscle.**

The inguinal canal runs between layers of the aponeuroses in the line of the inguinal ligament and marks the line of descent of the testis in the male. The sites where this enters and exits the canal comprise deficiencies in the abdominal wall through which a hernia may protrude.

The rectus abdominis muscles originate from the pubic bone inferiorly and insert into the xiphoid and medial costal cartilages.

Deep to these muscles and aponeuroses lies extraperitoneal fat and the peritoneum itself.

The layers are well seen with ultrasound, CT and MRI but are seldom imaged specifically other than in relation to intra-abdominal or pelvic pathology. Clinically, they are clearly important in abdominal and pelvic surgical practice, when the method for dividing them and repairing them is dictated by the access needed and the anatomy.

Applied Radiological Anatomy for Medical Students. Paul Butler, Adam Mitchell, and Harold Ellis (eds.) Published by Cambridge University Press. © P. Butler, A. Mitchell, and H. Ellis 2007.

The gastrointestinal tract

The gastrointestinal tract is a long tubular structure extending from the pharynx to the anal canal. There are many ways in which this can be imaged. Gas within bowel is visible on plain radiographs, while examinations using a suspension of barium sulfate to coat or fill the lumen demonstrate the anatomy and details of the bowel wall. CT and MRI can be used to study the cross-sectional anatomy and the surrounding anatomical structures. Less commonly, nuclear medicine techniques investigate functional anatomy, and, particularly in the infant, ultrasound has a role in studying the gut. Endoluminal ultrasound shows detailed wall structure and is used particularly in the assessment of tumors.

Esophagus

The esophagus is a muscular tube, around 23 cm long in the adult, extending from the level of C6 where it begins below the pharynx, to the gastro-esophageal junction at around T10. The majority of its course is within the thorax.

At its origin it is a flattened tube lying slightly to the left of the midline behind the trachea, with the prevertebral muscles posteriorly. Anterolaterally are the thyroid lobes and carotid arteries, and internal jugular veins, as well as the vagus nerves. The recurrent laryngeal nerves lie between it and the trachea.

Throughout the thoracic course of the esophagus, the vertebral column forms the major posterior relation, with the azygos and hemi-azygos venous systems to the right and left posteriorly and the thoracic duct between it and the azygos vein. The pleura lies close to it laterally on the right, other than where the azygos vein arches anteriorly to join the superior vena cava. On the left, the left subclavian artery and thoracic duct pass between it and the pleura in the superior mediastinum, and below this the aortic arch and descending thoracic aorta make up its main relations. From superior to inferior its anterior relations are the trachea, left main bronchus, and lymph nodes. Below this lie the pericardium and the left atrium and inferiorly the diaphragm.

It enters the abdomen between the left crus of the diaphragm and the left lobe of the liver and passes to the left of the midline towards the gastro-esophageal junction.

The blood supply of the esophagus derives from the inferior thyroid arteries in the neck, via small branches directly from the aorta in the thorax and from the celiac artery via the left gastric in its lower third. Its lymphatic drainage is to local nodes along its length, which drain superiorly into the deep cervical nodes and inferiorly towards the celiac axis group.

The muscular wall is skeletal muscle in the upper third with transition into smooth muscle in the lower third.

When distended with barium, the anterior wall of the oesophagus is indented by the arch of the aorta and inferiorly the left main bronchus. In the lower thorax the left atrium makes a long shallow anterior indentation in it (Fig. 5.2). Using barium and gas distension ("double contrast") the mucosa of the esophagus is demonstrated, and liquid and solid swallows allow dynamic assessment of motility. Motility is frequently studied with video series in the upper esophagus with the patient erect, whereas the lower esophagus is best assessed with the patient prone. CT and MRI allow visualization of the wall of the esophagus and the surrounding structures (Fig. 5.3). Endoscopic ultrasound gives very detailed information of the esophageal wall as well as of surrounding structures particularly local lymph nodes. This

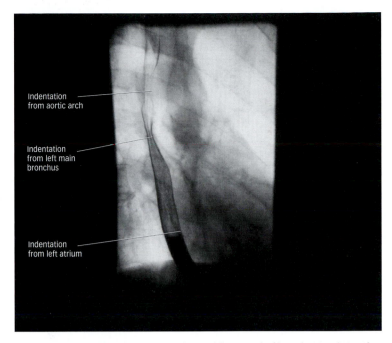

Fig. 5.2. **Barium swallow image taken in an oblique projection. The esophagus is outlined by barium and distended with air. Note shallow indentations form the arch of the aorta, the left main bronchus and, inferiorly, the left atrium.**

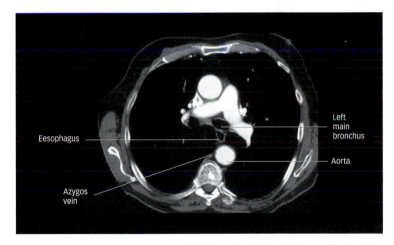

Fig. 5.3. **CT image to demonstrate the relations of the oesophagus in the mediastinum. Note the left main bronchus anteriorly and the aorta and azygous vein posteriorly. The pleura and lungs are the lateral relations.**

technique is almost exclusively used in the assessment of esophageal tumors and their local spread.

Stomach

The stomach is a wide muscular bag and represents the widest part of the gut. It has a variable shape and lie depending on the build of the subject. As well as having a roughly "J" shape in the erect position, its proximal part lies posteriorly, with the distal stomach curving anteriorly as it passes downwards and to the right. In the empty state it is flattened antero-posteriorly. The inferior edge is referred to as the greater curve, and the superior edge is the lesser curve. Inferiorly on the lesser curve is a variably defined notch called the incisura angularis.

The stomach is divided into a number of areas for the purposes of description, although these anatomical divisions are not strictly defined by changes in structure or function.

Proximally, the gastro-esophageal junction opens at the cardia into the fundus. This is the superior part and lies beneath the left hemidiaphragm. It also represents the most posterior part of the stomach. The body of the stomach extends from the fundus to the incisura where it then becomes the antrum. The pylorus or pyloric canal represents the outlet of the stomach into the duodenum and lies to the right of the midline at a variable level depending on gastric filling and position of the subject.

The wall of the stomach contains layered smooth muscle, while the mucosal surface contains large longitudinal mucosal folds called rugae. These become less prominent when the stomach is distended.

The anatomical relations of the stomach are anteriorly, the left lobe of the liver above and the abdominal wall inferiorly. Posterior to the stomach is a blind ended peritoneal recess called the lesser sac (see section on peritoneal anatomy) which lies between it and its posterior relations. These are the fibers of the left hemidiapragm arching upwards towards the dome of the diaphragm, the spleen, and splenic artery, the left adrenal and upper pole of the left kidney and, inferiorly the body and tail of pancreas overlaid by the transverse mesocolon.

The stomach is invested in peritoneum. This is in contact above the stomach to form the lesser omentum and, inferiorly, meets further folds of peritoneum from around the transverse colon to form the greater omentum, which often contains prominent fatty tissue and spreads inferiorly as an apron-like fold and is the first structure seen on opening the peritoneum anteriorly.

The blood supply is from branches of the celiac artery. The major branches run along the greater and lesser curves, small branches radiating from these over the anterior and posterior surface of the stomach.

The lymphatics correspond to the arterial branches, most draining to celiac axis groups.

The modalities used to image the stomach are as for the esophagus. Gas frequently makes the fundus particularly visible on the erect chest radiograph, while the body is often seen on the supine abdominal image. Double contrast barium techniques show the rugae and mucosa (Fig. 5.4), although the barium meal examination has been superseded in much clinical practice by endoscopy. In the infant, the pylorus may be evaluated by ultrasound in the diagnosis of infantile hypertrophic pyloric stenosis. Gastric emptying can be evaluated in a quantitative functional manner with isotope studies. CT is used in the evaluation of gastric malignancies, and the stomach's relations are well demonstrated on this and MRI (Fig. 5.5).

Duodenum

The duodenum is a roughly C-shaped tube, which runs from the pyloric canal to the jejunum. For most of its curved course it has the pancreas on its inner margin. For descriptive purposes it is divided into four parts, although there is no structural change between each part.

The first part of the duodenum passes posterosuperiorly from the pylorus. It is partly within the peritoneum but distally becomes retroperitoneal as is the rest of the duodenum. It is distensible on barium studies and is known as the duodenal cap. It has the posterior surface of the liver and the gall bladder as anterior and superior

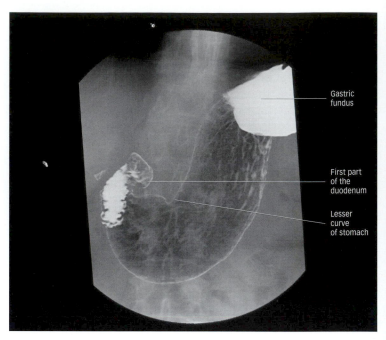

Fig. 5.4. **Stomach on barium meal, in supine position. The stomach mucosa is coated with barium and distended with air. The posteriorly-lying fundus contains dense barium. The first part of the duodenum is distended with air, while the descending second part contains barium.**

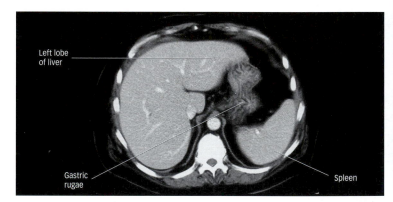

Fig. 5.5. **Axial CT image through the upper abdomen. The gastric rugae are well demonstrated (compare with the barium meal image). Note the position of the stomach, passing anteriorly below the left lobe of the liver, and on the anteromedial side of the spleen. Fat lying between these structures appears black on CT.**

relations. Posteriorly are the portal vein and bile duct, and the inferior vena cava. The gastroduodenal branch of the hepatic artery also lies posterior to it. On its inferior surface lies the pancreatic head.

The second part runs in a vertical orientation. On its medial surface lies the head of the pancreas and it is into it that the common bile duct and pancreatic duct open, usually together at the ampulla of Vater, but with common anatomical variations. Posteriorly lie the right renal vessels, renal pelvis, and part of the kidney itself. Anteriorly and laterally lie parts of the colon (the hepatic flexure and proximal transverse colon) and part of the right lobe of the liver.

The third part of the duodenum is the longest and most posterior. It lies horizontally and crosses the midline from right to left. The pancreas is superior to it. It passes behind the superior mesenteric vessels and anterior to the aorta and inferior vena cava. The superior mesenteric vessels enter the root of the small bowel mesentery which passes across its anterior surface.

The shortest part of the duodenum is the fourth part which passes superiorly and to the left. It lies on the psoas muscle and left side of the aorta and loops of small bowel lie anterior to it. It becomes jejunum where it emerges from the retroperitoneum at the level of L2.

The duodenum receives its blood supply from branches of the celiac artery, mainly via the gastroduodenal branch, and from branches of the superior mesenteric artery. These arteries give rise to a network of small vessels supplying the duodenum and pancreas.

Barium studies (Fig. 5.6) and cross sectional imaging (Fig. 5.7) are the main radiological tools used for studying the duodenum. Endoscopy has replaced barium for much of its investigation.

Jejunum and ileum

The jejunum and ileum comprise the most important part of the alimentary tract for absorption of nutrients and form the longest section. The transition from jejunum to ileum is a gradual one, the jejunum being the initial two-fifths of this length of bowel. There are differences in the arterial anatomy from jejunum to ileum, and

differences in the appearance of the mucosal fold pattern. The mucosal folds (valvulae conniventes) are more prominent in the jejunum becoming less visible or even absent towards the distal ileum. The jejunum is slightly wider than the ileum (2.5 cm vs. 2 cm). The loops are convoluted and coiled within the peritoneal cavity and anchored by the small bowel mesentery to the posterior abdominal wall. The root of this mesentery runs inferiorly and across the midline from the duodenojejunal flexure on the left side, to the right lower part of the posterior abdominal wall overlying the right sacroiliac joint. This mesentery consists of two layers of peritoneum within which run the vessels supplying the small and much of the large bowel and lymphatics as well as some fat. As the small intestine is so convoluted, this fan-like mesentery has a similarly folded appearance. The blood supply is via the superior mesenteric artery, the branches of which radiate out within the mesentery. The venous drainage and lymphatic drainage is within the mesentery also.

The anterior relation is the transverse colon and the greater omentum. The posterior relation is peritoneum overlying the structures within the retroperitoneum.

Radiologically, as with the rest of the gut, barium studies are commonly used to investigate the small bowel (Fig. 5.8). This can be drunk by the patient as a barium follow-through, or introduced via a nasojejunal tube as a small bowel enema (enteroclysis). Particularly in cases of bowel obstruction, gas is seen within the small intestine on plain radiographs of the abdomen. CT and MRI investigate the small bowel and its relationship to other organs (Fig. 5.9), and both of these cross-sectional techniques can be employed with contrast in the bowel lumen to produce cross-sectional images.

Ultrasound may show small bowel pathology particularly when there is an obstruction or free peritoneal fluid, and radionuclide scans are also used to assess inflammation in inflammatory bowel disease, or ectopic gastric mucosa in a Meckel's diverticulum (an embryological remnant) which may produce bleeding into the gut.

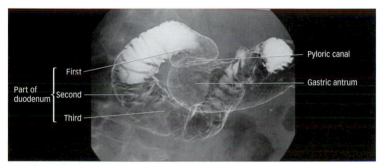

Fig. 5.6. **Duodenum on barium meal. Barium coats the mucosa with its characteristic mucosal folds, and it is partly distended with gas. The short pyloric canal accounts for the constriction between the gastric antrum and the well-distended first part of the duodenum.**

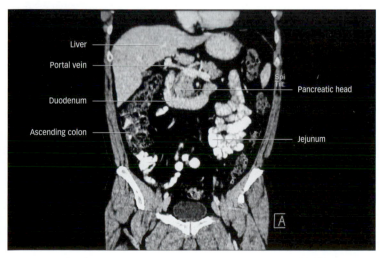

Fig. 5.7. **The second, third, and fourth part of the duodenum are seen here on a coronal reconstruction from an axial CT scan. Lying on the inside of the curve formed by the duodenum is the pancreatic head and the portal vein passes obliquely towards the liver.**

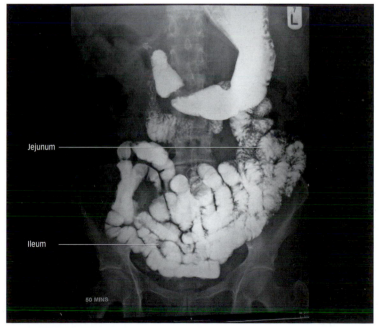

Fig. 5.8. **Small intestine on barium follow-through. Barium remains in the stomach.**

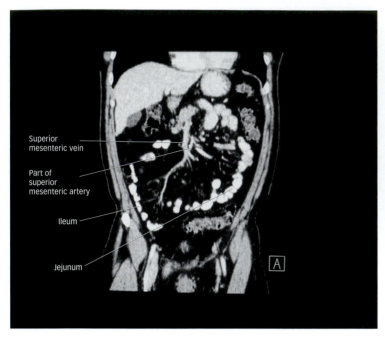

Fig. 5.9. **Small intestine on a coronal CT reformat. Note the similarity with the small bowel barium study. Some of the mesenteric vessels passing in the mesentery (fat within mesentery here is black) are well shown (compare these with the angiographic images elsewhere in this book).**

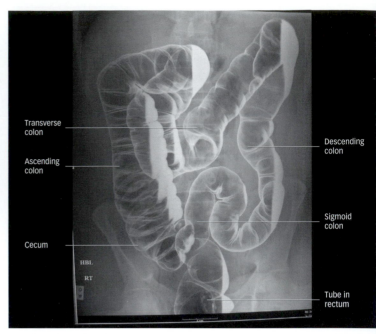

Fig. 5.10. **Whole colon demonstrated on barium enema. White barium coats the mucosa and the lumen is distended with gas. This image is taken with the patient lying on the left side, accounting for the fluid levels. There is variation in the length of the colon and the configuration of the non fixed parts (transverse and sigmoid colon).**

Colon (including rectum)

The large bowel connects the terminal ileum to the anal canal. It consists of the cecum, in the right iliac fossa, the ascending colon, the transverse colon extending from the hepatic flexure on the right to the splenic flexure in the left upper quadrant. From the left upper quadrant, the descending colon passes inferiorly to the sigmoid colon, thence the rectum and anal canal (Fig. 5.10).

The cecum is that portion of the right side of the colon inferior to the ileocecal valve where the terminal ileum enters the large bowel. It is a blind-ended sac, which is the widest part of the large bowel and into it enters the vermiform appendix. The cecum is a variable length and is usually covered anteriorly and on each side by peritoneum, but this does not completely surround it. There is some variability in this and the cecum may be long and completely intraperitoneal. The appendix has its own mesentery (the meso-appendix) in which runs its own artery. The length and position of the appendix is quite variable; it may be retrocaecal and pass superiorly, or extend inferiorly into the true pelvis. The ileocecal valve is variable in its appearance and may protrude into the lumen of the cecum or be flat.

The ascending colon extends superiorly to the hepatic flexure. It is retroperitoneal, the peritoneal reflection on its lateral side forming a shallow potential channel called the right paracolic gutter. The hepatic flexure usually lies below the right lobe of the liver.

The transverse colon (Fig. 5.11) is invested by layers of peritoneum and is bowed anteriorly and inferiorly. In some subjects it may have a long inferior loop extending into the pelvis. The peritoneal surfaces around the transverse colon anchor it to the posterior abdominal wall as the transverse mesocolon. The peritoneum surrounding the stomach and first part of the duodenum extends inferiorly to join that around the transverse colon and together these form the greater omentum (described above).

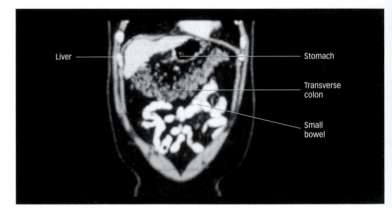

Fig. 5.11. **Coronal reformat CT showing the transverse colon. Note the stomach and liver superiorly and small bowel loops inferiorly.**

The splenic flexure is where the colon once more becomes retroperitoneal. From the phrenicocolic ligament beneath the left hemidiaphragm, the descending colon passes inferiorly. At the pelvic brim it becomes the sigmoid colon, a variable length of colon, which is once more intraperitoneal, with its own mesocolon, the root of which lies over the left sacroiliac joint and sacrum in an inverted V-shape. As this becomes the rectum, the peritoneum is confined to its anterior and lateral surfaces in the upper third, over some of its anterior surface in the mid rectum. Inferiorly it is below the peritoneal cavity. It joins the anal canal at the floor of the true pelvis.

The cecum, ascending and descending colon lie anterior and lateral to their respective psoas muscles and femoral nerves as well as to the muscles of the posterior abdominal wall. Laterally lie the iliolumbar ligaments and origins of the transversus abdominis muscles. More inferiorly, the colon lies anterior to the iliac bones and the iliacus muscles. The anterior relations of each side are similar, being mainly loops of small bowel and the lateral part of the anterior abdominal wall. The splenic flexure lies inferior to the spleen and lower slips of the left hemidiaphragm, the hepatic flexure is usually beneath the right lobe of the liver, although it may interpose between this and the right hemidiaphragm.

The transverse colon is the first structure encountered with the greater omentum on opening the peritoneum. Posterior to it lie small bowel loops, and the second part of the duodenum, and a part of the pancreatic head.

The sigmoid colon is variable in length (Fig. 5.12) and the relations will be dictated by this and the state of bladder filling. The bladder and uterus in the female lie inferiorly and anteriorly to it and, for the most part elsewhere, it is bordered by loops of ileum. Posteriorly lies its mesentery, the sacrum and rectum.

The rectum is bordered posteriorly by the sacrum and coccyx, the origins of muscles of the pelvic floor, and sympathetic nerves. Anteriorly lie the peritoneal reflection and small bowel and sigmoid colon superiorly, then the seminal vesicles, vas deferens, bladder, and prostate in the male, and the vagina, cervix, and uterus in the female.

The blood supply of the large bowel is derived from the superior mesenteric artery as far as the distal transverse colon and thereafter via branches of the inferior mesenteric artery. These are discussed elsewhere. Lymphatics drain along the lines of the arteries.

Gas in the colon is usually appreciated on a plain abdominal radiograph. It can be imaged with barium and air in a double contrast barium enema to give mucosal detail after strong purgative laxatives have emptied it of stool (Figs. 5.10, 5.12), or with a water-soluble single contrast enema simply to demonstrate a level if obstruction is suspected. During a barium enema, the patient is moved on the examination couch to allow coating of the entire colon and optimal demonstration of the length of the colon in different projections to separate overlapping loops (although in a long tortuous bowel this may be difficult). On a barium enema, the folds of the colon wall (haustra) are demonstrated readily. These are sometimes less prominent within the lower descending colon and sigmoid.

The ileocecal valve is usually identifiable as a filling defect on the posteromedial wall of the cecum. The appendix often fills with barium or air.

When insufflated with air, a CT scan can give detail of the bowel wall also (CT pneumocolon) and both CT and MRI may allow assess-

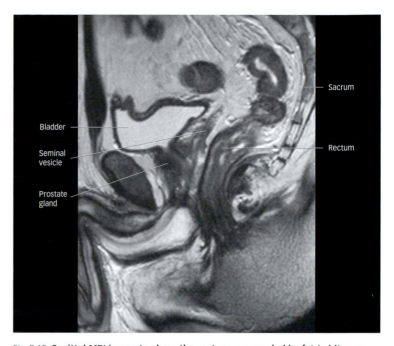

Fig. 5.13. **Sagittal MRI image to show the rectum surrounded by fat (white on this sequence) and small vessels anteriorly to the sacrum and posterior to the seminal vesicles, bladder and prostate in this male patient. Note also the angle at the ano-rectal junction.**

ment of the wall and the relationship of pathology to surrounding structures (Fig. 5.11).

In cases of colonic bleeding, angiography may be used to assess for a bleeding point, or radionuclide scans may be used if the bleeding is less acute. Ultrasound may be used to assess for suspected appendicitis and occasionally is used to observe sites of bowel wall thickening.

The rectum being relatively fixed is well evaluated with MRI (Fig. 5.13) particularly to investigate rectal tumors.

Anal canal

The anal canal (Fig. 5.14) represents the final part of the alimentary tract. It is a short (around 3 cm) tubular canal surrounded by the internal and external anal sphincter. At its junction with the rectum, the puborectalis muscle loops posteriorly around it making the anorectal junction of around 90 degrees. From this point, the anal canal runs posteriorly and inferiorly to the anal verge.

The internal sphincter is continuous with the circular muscle of the rectum, while the external sphincter superiorly is continuous with the levator ani muscles of the pelvic floor. More inferiorly, it comprises a muscle sling, that runs from the perineal body to the tip of the coccyx, and below this circular fibers completely surround the canal. These three components of the sphincter are often not separated clearly from each other, and are under voluntary control. The arterial supply to the anal canal is from the superior rectal artery and inferiorly from the inferior rectal artery. The lymphatic drainage is important. Superiorly, the lymphatic channels drain to internal iliac nodes, while the lower anal canal drains to the inguinal nodes. This division is a function of the anal canal marking the junction between the embryonic hindgut and the skin surface of the perineum.

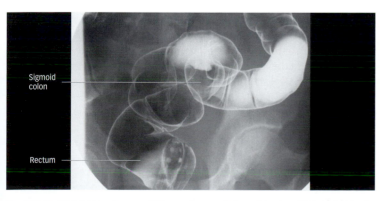

Fig. 5.12. **Barium enema image of the rectum and sigmoid colon. Note the tube in the rectum. This view is taken obliquely.**

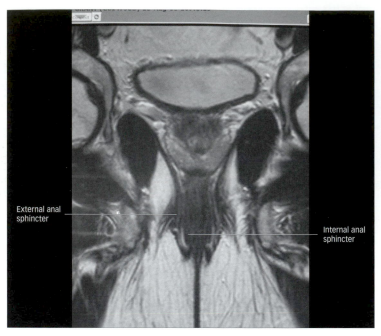

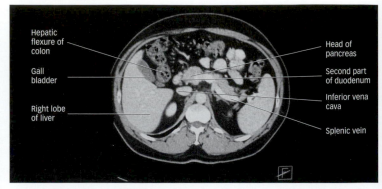

Fig. 5.15. **Axial CT image through the right lobe of the liver at the level of the gall bladder. At this level also lies much of the head and body of the pancreas and the spleen. The splenic vein is well seen posterior to the tail of pancreas.**

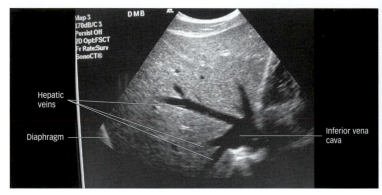

Fig. 5.16. **Ultrasound image through the liver superiorly. The hepatic veins are seen as black tubular structures converging on the inferior vena cava. The heart lies to the right of the image.**

Fig. 5.14. **Oblique Coronal MRI image through the anal canal. The thin external sphincter muscle laterally surrounds thicker internal sphincter. Laterally lies the ischio-anal fat, superiorly is the prostate gland and bladder.**

Below the pelvic floor muscles, the anal canal is surrounded by fat. The pyramidal-shaped fat deposits on each side are called ischiorectal fossae.

Imaging of the anal canal itself is not commonly performed as it can be viewed directly from the mucosal surface. Imaging is used in the investigation of sphincter damage (most commonly following birth trauma) when MRI or endoluminal ultrasound are used most commonly, and in the investigation of perianal abscesses and fistulae to plan the surgery needed to drain these effectively. CT is employed to assess spread of anal tumors and MRI can also be used for this.

Liver

The liver is the largest solid organ and has complex anatomy. It is very commonly the subject of imaging investigations as it is affected by spread of tumors, as well as having its own range of diseases.

Ultrasound is usually the initial investigation (Fig. 5.15) and is useful to categorize liver disease, suspected on blood tests, into disease affecting the drainage of bile from the liver via the bile ducts, or disease affecting the liver parenchyma itself. If disease is obstructing the bile ducts, further investigations may involve injecting iodinated contrast agents into the biliary tree. This can be performed via an endoscope in the duodenum, with access to the biliary tree via the ampulla of Vater (endoscopic retrograde cholangiopancreatogram (ERCP)), or alternatively the bile ducts within the liver can be punctured through the wall of the abdomen and the liver tissue (percutaneous transhepatic cholangiogram (PTC)). Magnetic resonance imaging can also be used to show the ducts and this is less invasive than the other techniques. Oral or intravenous agents which are excreted into the bile have been used to show these on CT or plain radiographs, but this is largely superseded by newer techniques.

To investigate the liver tissue itself, CT (Fig. 5.16) or MRI are frequently used, and these will show focal abnormalities against the background of the normal liver tissue. Injections of contrast agents into the bloodstream are commonly used to accentuate the differences between the normal and abnormal liver tissue. Some of these demonstrate differences in the blood supply to the different tissues, while some are taken up within liver tissue or tumor and therefore allow differentiation of normal from abnormal areas. Ultrasound has also been used recently with contrast agents with similar aims.

Liver diseases often produce variations in the flow of blood into or out of the liver and can be imaged with arteriography or hepatic venography. Much of this information can now be shown with CT or MRI. Information on flow and its direction and velocity can be shown with doppler ultrasound, and during operations on the liver, the ultrasound probe may be placed directly onto the surface of the liver.

Nuclear medicine techniques also exist for evaluating the functional anatomy of the liver using agents excreted into the bile or taken up by the liver tissue.

Anatomy

The liver has a smooth anterior and superior surface, which has a relatively straight lower border from deep to the lower left costal margin across the midline running inferiorly and to the right deep to the right costal margin to the lateral abdominal wall. Most of it is therefore deep to ribs and costal cartilages. The posterior and inferior surface is irregular and borders numerous other intrabdominal structures. The liver is sometimes described as containing four lobes: right, left, quadrate, and caudate. For planning surgery, a segmental anatomical description is used based on segments bordered by the main portal vein branches and the three main hepatic veins. This seems initially complex, but less so once the plains of this division are appreciated.

Key to the liver anatomy is the fact that it has a dual blood supply: arterial blood accounts for around 10% to 20% of its blood supply and the portal vein providing the rest. This vein carries nutrient-rich blood from the gut and is much larger than the hepatic artery. The artery and portal vein branches run with the bile ducts taking bile in the opposite direction towards the duodenum. The hepatic veins drain directly into the inferior vena cava (Fig. 5.15). Usually there are three main veins (right, middle, and left) entering the vena cava immediately below the diaphragm, close to the right atrium, and a smaller one draining only segment 1 (caudate). In conditions restricting flow of blood through the portal circulation (including cirrhosis of the liver), portal venous blood may enter the systemic circulation via collateral vessels which enlarge. These are commonly seen in the lower esophagus as varices, or within the anterior abdominal wall where these can be visible around the umbilicus. Such portosystemic anastomoses may also be seen in the anal canal and around the hilum of the spleen and left kidney.

The smooth anterior surface is related to the inner aspect of ribs and costal margins, the inferior posterior surface is related to the esophagus and stomach on the left, and on the right to the gall bladder, the second part of the duodenum, the hepatic flexure of the colon and the right kidney, and adrenal gland.

The site where the artery and portal vein enter the liver, and the common hepatic duct (draining bile) exits the liver, is referred to as the hepatic hilum. These structures then run in the hepatoduodenal ligament towards the duodenum and pancreatic head. This is in a fold of peritoneum behind which is the entrance to the lesser sac (see peritoneum section).

Entering the anterior surface of the liver is the obliterated umbilical vein, which extends from the anterior abdominal wall within the free edge of the falciform ligament. This fissure within the anterior surface is an easily identifiable landmark on imaging. The peritoneal reflections are described in the appropriate section.

Gall bladder

This blind-ended sac is an outpouching from the biliary system. It lies immediately beneath the inferior surface of the liver (below segment 4b, the quadrate lobe) in which it produces a smooth indentation. It is around 10 cm long and connected to the common hepatic duct by the cystic duct. The confluence of these gives rise to the common bile duct. The fundus of the gall bladder lies close to, or against, the anterior abdominal wall at the point where the lateral margin of the rectus abdominis muscle meets the right costal margin.

The gall bladder is most commonly evaluated with ultrasound (Fig. 5.17), and gall stones or inflammatory thickening are easily appreciated. It is usually covered on its inferior surface with peritoneum although this may surround it completely. Further variations exist for much of the gall bladder anatomy, including variation in the relationship of the cystic duct to the hepatic artery, the length and insertion

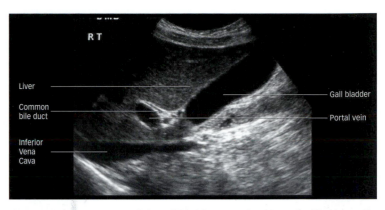

Fig. 5.17. **Ultrasound image of the gall bladder. Note the thin wall. It lies beneath the liver.**

of the cystic duct, the origin of the cystic artery (usually from the right hepatic artery). These are important for laparoscopic gall bladder surgery when their appreciation is vital to avoid complications.

The inferior relations of the gall bladder are the second part of the duodenum and hepatic flexure of the colon.

Spleen

The spleen is a vascular organ located under the left hemidiaphragm. In normal adults it measures around 12 cm in maximum length and, like the liver, it has a curved superior and lateral surface lying against the diaphragm and overlain by the lower ribs, and an inferomedial surface bearing impressions from its anatomical relations. These are the kidney posteroinferiorly, the splenic flexure of the colon anteriorly, and the gastric fundus posteromedially. Centrally in its inferior surface, the tail of the pancreas lies in contact with it. The anterior surface has a notch between the gastric and colic areas, which can be easily palpable when the spleen enlarges significantly.

The spleen is surrounded by peritoneum. Two layers from the posterior abdominal wall separate to surround it, and rejoin at the splenic hilum from where they continue to surround the stomach. These layers form the gastrosplenic ligament.

The splenic artery is a large tortuous branch of the celiac artery, which runs superior to the body and tail of pancreas to enter the spleen at its hilum. The splenic vein exits the hilum and runs posterior to the tail and body of the pancreas, forming the portal vein at its union with the superior mesenteric vein. There are numerous potential collateral channels that can drain splenic venous blood if the portal flow is reduced in liver disease and these drain into the venous systems of neighboring organs, most commonly the gastric fundus and lower esophagus, and the renal vein.

The spleen is easily seen with ultrasound in most individuals, but in some cases CT (Fig. 5.16) or MRI are used to assess perfusion and the vessels, especially following trauma to the lower chest when rib fractures may also be present. Rarely, arteriography is used if there is disease affecting the blood supply, and an injection into the artery allows a delayed image to show the venous drainage and the portal vein. White cells labelled with radio-isotopes can also be used to assess splenic function.

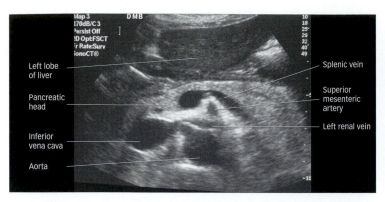

Left lobe of liver · Pancreatic head · Inferior vena cava · Aorta · Splenic vein · Superior mesenteric artery · Left renal vein

Cystic duct · Common bile duct · Gall bladder · Intrahepatic bile ducts · Pancreatic duct

Fig. 5.18. Transverse ultrasound image of the left lobe of the liver and pancreas. The stomach is collapsed and accounts for the thin black lines between them. The light gray pancreas can be seen curving around the black vessels of the splenic vein and the beginning of the portal vein. Behind this lie the inferior vena cava and the aorta.

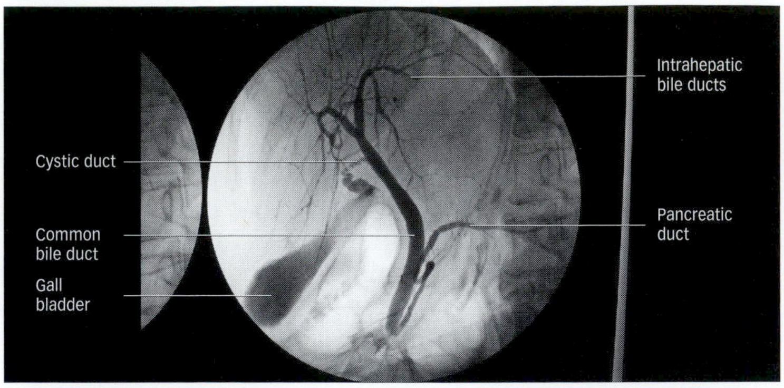

Fig. 5.19. ERCP image showing the intrahepatic biliary tree, the common bile duct. The cystic duct, which is characteristically tortuous, runs from the gall bladder. The pancreatic duct is also opacified. On this view the patient is oblique, which accounts for the apparent "loop" of the pancreatic duct as it passes towards the X-ray detector.

Pancreas

The pancreas is a non-encapsulated retroperitoneal organ with exocrine and endocrine function. It lies in the upper abdomen and contains a variable amount of fat between lobules of tissue. It tapers in size from the pancreatic head to the right of the midline, into a thinner neck, body, and tail, which run obliquely to the left, superiorly, and posteriorly. The endocrine portion comprises the Islets of Langerhans, and these cannot be shown by standard imaging techniques. Most imaging is performed to investigate pathology relating to the exocrine gland, its duct, and anatomically related structures.

The pancreas is variably seen with ultrasound due to the presence of overlying gas. When well seen this is a good modality for assessing it; however, CT and MRI are more reliably able to demonstrate it, as well as allowing assessment of its perfusion. Nuclear medicine techniques are used particularly in the assessment of endocrine tumours of the pancreas by labelling, with radio-isotopes, chemical precursors to the hormones they produce. Assessment of the pancreatic duct in conditions such as chronic pancreatitis can be made via direct cannulation of it at endoscopy (endoscopic retrograde pancreatography) (Fig. 5.19), although magnetic resonance imaging can also give some of this information.

The head of the pancreas lies on the inside of the curve formed by the first three parts of the duodenum. The superior mesenteric artery and vein run posterior to this, the vein being joined by the splenic vein to form the portal vein which then ascends behind the head and neck to the right, obliquely towards the liver. The uncinate process of the pancreas is the most inferior and posterior portion and hooks medially from the head, behind the mesenteric vessels which are thus surrounded by pancreatic tissue anteriorly, on the right and posteriorly.

In the same direction as the portal vein, the hepatic artery passes towards the liver and the common bile duct transmits bile from the liver and gall bladder towards the duodenum. These three important tubular structures make an important landmark running parallel to each other between the pancreatic head and the hepatic hilum.

The pancreatic duct extends from the tail to the head of the gland and opens into the second part of the duodenum with the common bile duct at the ampulla of Vater. There are a number of anatomical variation owing to the gland's embryology (it is formed by the fusion of two separate buds, whose ducts fuse variably). The most important point is that a second more superior opening into the duodenum may drain the majority of the gland, with a smaller contribution from the lower, more typical duct opening.

The relations of the pancreas are anteriorly the lesser sac of the peritoneum, which is a potential space between it, and the posterior wall of the stomach. Superiorly and anteriorly lies the left lobe of the liver. Posteriorly lie the splenic vein, the superior mesenteric vessels, the aorta, and inferior vena cava and on the right, the portal vein and hepatic artery, and bile duct. The body and tail overlie the upper part of the left kidney and the tail extends towards the splenic hilum. The main lateral relation of the head is the duodenum. Most of these anatomical relations are separated from it by variable amounts of retroperitoneal fat. In thin patients this may be almost completely absent, but in some cases there may be many centimeters separating it from adjacent structures.

The pancreas receives its blood supply from branches of the coeliac artery via the splenic and hepatic arteries. The main named branches are the pancreatica magna from the splenic artery and the gastroduodenal artery from the hepatic. This forms anastomoses around the head and uncinate with arterial contributions from the superior mesenteric artery. The venous drainage is similarly into splenic vein, superior mesenteric vein and portal vein. Local lymph nodes, analogous to the arterial supply, drain towards coeliac nodes.

Peritoneum and peritoneal spaces

The peritoneum is the enveloping membrane, which encloses the intra-abdominal organs. It is essentially a closed sac, between the outer boundaries of the abdominal and pelvic cavity and the organs contained within.

The parietal peritoneum is the outer surface, which lies deep to the abdominal wall muscles, beneath the diaphragm, above the pelvic organs and anterior to the structures of the retroperitoneum posteriorly.

The visceral peritoneum is the complex, folded surface, which encloses most of the organs within the abdominal cavity.

In health, the peritoneal cavity contains only a small volume of fluid enabling the structures to move freely over each other with respiration, movement and gut peristalsis. There is usually slightly more fluid within the peritoneum in females (and the Fallopian tubes open into the peritoneum, as the only site where the surface is incomplete).

The intra-abdominal alimentary tract lies within the peritoneal cavity for the most part, but most of the duodenum and the ascending and descending colon lie in the retroperitoneum. The rectum is covered anteriorly by peritoneum in its upper third. More inferiorly, it passes beneath the pelvic reflection of the peritoneum.

The vessels passing to abdominal organs lie within folds of peritoneum known as mesenteries. Where two layers of peritoneum pass from the parietal surface to surrounding organs, these are called ligaments or omenta. These are of variable length and serve to anchor the abdominal contents to different extents. For example, the mesentery containing vessels and lymphatics passing to the small bowel is long, allowing for the necessary changes in position during peristalsis and following meals, while the short reflections of peritoneum from the diaphragm onto the liver keep this organ relatively fixed in position as is also the case for the spleen.

Because of its complex folded nature, and because the gut passes in several places from retroperitoneum to intraperitoneal position, there are a large number or recesses or blind-ended sacs. Many of these have names, but it must be remembered that, unless there is inflammation causing these to be walled off, or following surgery, the whole peritoneal cavity is continuous, and material flows freely within it tending to track towards the pelvic reflections as a result of gravity, and toward the subphrenic spaces (beneath the diaphragms), as these develop a small negative pressure during respiration.

The most clinically important recesses of peritoneum

Subphrenic spaces
These are where it reflects onto the spleen and liver (although a small area of the liver is in direct contact with the right hemidiaphragm, known as the bare area) (Fig. 5.20).

Lesser sac
This lies between the posterior surface of the stomach and the anterior surface of the pancreas and is a blind-ended sac, communicating with

the main cavity behind the vessels running towards the liver hilum from the second part of the duodenum. This small communication is called the epiploic foramen (of Winslow). This sac can accumulate fluid when the pancreas has been inflamed (Fig. 5.20).

Subhepatic space
This is in free communication with the main peritoneal cavity, but may be a site of local fluid accumulation in gall bladder disease.

Pelvic recesses
The uterovesical pouch is the pelvic recess between bladder and uterus in the female, and the rectouterine pouch (also known as the pouch of Douglas) lies posteriorly and is frequently seen to contain fluid in inflammatory or malignant disease affecting the peritoneum (Fig. 5.21).

The most important ligaments and omenta

Greater omentum
An apron-like fold of several layers of peritoneum extending inferiorly from the greater curve of the stomach and the transverse colon, often for a considerable distance. This frequently contains much fat and is the first structure seen once the abdominal cavity is opened at surgery.

Lesser omentum
These are the two layers from the inferior surface of the liver to the lesser curve of the stomach.

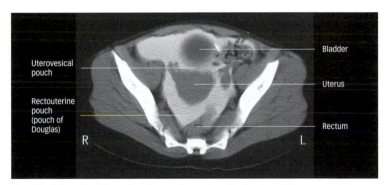

Fig. 5.21. **Axial CT with contrast in peritoneal cavity to show the paravesical spaces, the uterovesical pouch, and the rectouterine pouch (pouch of Douglas).**

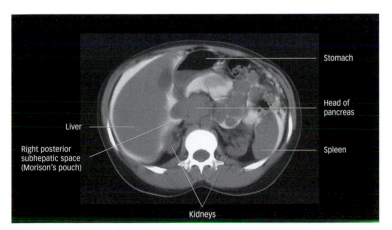

Fig. 5.20. **Axial CT with contrast in peritoneal cavity to show the anterior right subhepatic space, the posterior right subhepatic space (Morison's pouch), and the inferior recess of the lesser sac.**

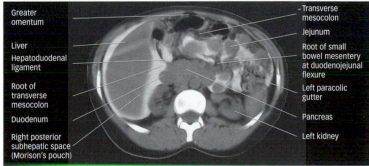

Fig. 5.22. **Axial CT with contrast in peritoneal cavity to show the root of the transverse mesocolon, the root of the small bowel mesentery, the greater omentum, and the duodenocolic ligament.**

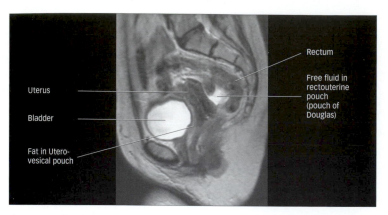

Fig. 5.23. **Sagittal MRI which shows free fluid in the rectouterine pouch (pouch of Douglas).**

Falciform ligament

This contains the obliterated umbilical vein and therefore runs from the umbilicus and anterior abdominal wall to a fissure on the anterior surface of the liver.

Coronary ligaments

These are the reflections of peritoneum onto the liver.

Transverse mesocolon and small bowel mesentery

These broad mesenteries fan out towards their respective parts of the gut and contain vessels and variable fat (Figs. 5.22, 5.23).

In health, the peritoneum is too thin to be demonstrable, but it can be thickened when inflamed, or infiltrated by tumors. Fluid within it makes its recesses and folds easy to demonstrate, and the folds and spaces are frequently referred to when assessing pathology within the abdominal cavity.

Section 3 | The abdomen and pelvis

Chapter 6 | The renal tract, retroperitoneum and pelvis

ANDREA G. ROCKALL
and SARAH J. VINNICOMBE

Imaging methods

The gross bony anatomy of the pelvis, as well as the detailed trabecular pattern of bone, is well demonstrated on conventional radiographs. CT provides superior three-dimensional spatial relationships, for example, in the demonstration of bone fragments in pelvic fractures or the position of a ureteric calculus. MRI provides unique information regarding bone marrow components such as fat, hemopoietic tissue, and bone marrow pathology. The soft tissues of the renal tract and pelvis are demonstrated using ultrasound, CT, and MRI, which all provide complementary information. Ultrasound and MRI have the advantage of not utilizing ionizing radiation. Ultrasound is the first imaging modality used to assess the kidneys and renal tract as a basic screen, due to its easy accessibility, lack of radiation, and low cost. In the pelvis, a full bladder is needed to act as an acoustic window and to displace gas-filled loops of bowel out of the pelvis. Endovaginal and transrectal ultrasound, though invasive, can provide exquisite detail of the internal anatomy of the female genital tract, male prostate and seminal vesicles without the necessity of a full bladder. MRI provides similar detail. The hysterosalpingogram (HSG) still has an important role in the evaluation of the uterine cavity and Fallopian tubes.

Arteriography and venography are the gold standards for demonstrating the vasculature of the retroperitoneum and pelvis, although MRI and contrast-enhanced CT (particularly multidetector CT) are used increasingly as non-invasive angiographic techniques.

The urinary tract is also investigated using iodinated contrast studies. These include the intravenous urogram (IVU) and the micturating cystourethrogram (MCUG). The former will normally demonstrate the pelvicalyceal systems, lower ureters, and the full bladder outline, whereas the MCUG demonstrates the entire urethra during micturition. Nuclear medicine techniques (scintigraphy) give important functional information on the renal tract.

The renal tract and retroperitoneum

The retroperitoneum is the space that lies posterior to the abdominal peritoneum and anterior to the muscles of the back. This space contains the following major structures:

- The kidneys and ureters
- The adrenal glands
- The abdominal aorta and inferior vena cava (IVC) and associated lymphatics
- The pancreas and part of the duodenum (see Chapter X)
- The posterior aspects of the ascending and descending colon (see Chapter X)
- The lumbosacral nerve plexus and sympathetic trunks.

The kidneys
Gross anatomy of the kidneys

The kidneys lie in the superior part of the retroperitoneum on either side of the vertebral column at approximately the levels of L1–L4. The right kidney usually lies slightly lower than the left, due to the bulk of the liver. The kidneys move up and down by 1–2 cm during deep inspiration and expiration. In the adult, the bipolar length of the kidney is usually approximately 11 cm. Discrepancy between right and left renal length of up to 1.5 cm is within normal limits. The upper poles of the kidneys lie more medial and posterior than the lower poles (Fig. 6.1). The kidneys are surrounded by a layer of fat, the perinephric fat, which is encapsulated by the perinephric fascia (Gerota's fascia) (Figs. 6.1 and 6.2).

Structure of the kidney

The kidney is covered by a fibrous capsule, which is closely applied to the renal cortex. The renal cortex forms the outer third of the kidney. Columns of cortex (columns of Bertin) extend medially into the medulla between the pyramids (Figs. 6.1 and 6.2). The renal medulla lies deep to the cortex and forms the inner two thirds. The medulla contains the renal pyramids, which are cone-shaped, with the apex (the papilla) pointing into the renal hilum (Fig. 6.1). The medullary rays run from the cortex into the papilla. Each papilla projects into the cup of a renal calyx, which drains via an infundibulum into the renal pelvis (Fig. 6.3). The renal pelvis is a funnel-shaped structure at the upper end of the ureter. It normally divides into two or three major calyces: the upper and lower pole calyces and in some cases

Applied Radiological Anatomy for Medical Students. Paul Butler, Adam Mitchell, and Harold Ellis (eds.) Published by Cambridge University Press. © P. Butler, A. Mitchell, and H. Ellis 2007.

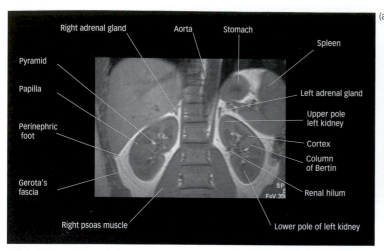

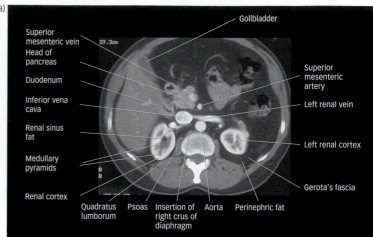

(a)

Fig. 6.1. **Coronal T1W MRI through the kidneys. The upper poles lie medial in relation to the lower poles. The renal cortex has an intermediate signal intensity and the medullary pyramids have a low signal intensity. The renal sinus fat is of high signal intensity.**

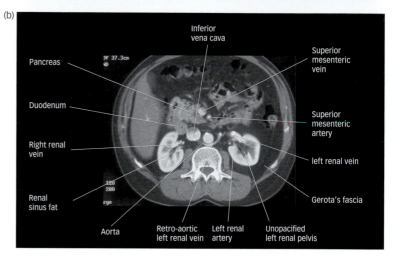

(b)

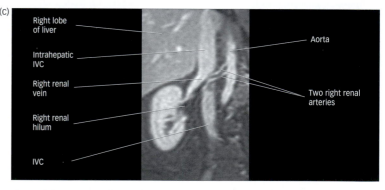

(c)

a third calyx between those at each pole (Fig. 6.3). Each major calyx then divides into two or three minor calyces, which have a cup-shape, indented by the apex of the accompanying renal pyramid. The renal hilum contains the renal pelvis, the renal artery, the renal vein and lymphatics, all of which are surrounded by renal sinus fat (Figs. 6.1 and 6.2).

Renal arteries, veins and lymphatic drainage

The right and left renal arteries arise from the abdominal aorta, at approximately the level of the superior margin of L2, immediately caudal to the origin of the superior mesenteric artery (see Fig. 6.22). There is usually a single artery supplying each kidney, although there are many anatomical variants, with up to four renal arteries supplying each kidney (Fig. 6.2c). The renal artery divides in the renal hilum into three branches. Two branches run anteriorly, supplying the anterior upper pole and entire lower pole, and one runs posteriorly supplying the posterior upper pole and mid pole.

Five or six veins arise within the kidney and join to form the renal vein, which runs anterior to the artery within the renal pelvis (Fig. 6.2). The right renal vein has a short course, running directly into the IVC. The left renal vein runs anterior to the abdominal aorta and then drains into the IVC. Occasionally, the left renal vein runs posterior to the aorta, known as a retro-aortic renal vein. The left renal vein receives tributaries from the left inferior phrenic vein, the left gonadal and the left adrenal vein.

The lymphatic drainage of the kidneys follows the renal arteries to nodes situated at the origin of the renal arteries in the para-aortic region.

Nerve supply

The sympathetic nerves supplying the kidney arise in the renal sympathetic plexus and run along the renal vessels. Afferent fibres, including pain fibers, travel with the sympathetic fibers through the splanchnic nerves and join the dorsal roots of the 11th and 12th thoracic and the 1st and 2nd lumbar levels.

Fig. 6.2. **(a) CT scan at the cortico-medullary phase, 40 seconds after administration of intravenous contrast medium. The renal cortex is brightly enhancing. The renal medulla is of lower attenuation. The aorta and its branches (superior mesenteric and renal arteries) are homogeneously enhanced. (b) CT scan at the cortico-medullary phase, just below Fig. 6.2 (a). Note the left renal vein passing posteriorly to the aorta (retro-aortic). The renal pelves are unopacified at this early stage following contrast administration. (c) MR venogram in the coronal plane demonstrates the right renal vein draining directly into the IVC. There are two right renal arteries, an anatomical variant.**

Fascial spaces around the kidney

The kidney is surrounded by perirenal fat, which is completely encircled by a fascial plane (Gerota's fascia), which also encases the suprarenal gland (Figs. 6.1 and 6.2). Medially, Gerota's fascia blends with the fascia surrounding the aorta and IVC.

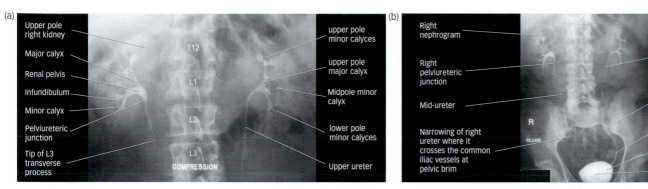

Fig. 6.3. **(a)** Intravenous urogram (compression view) demonstrating bilateral smooth nephrograms and opacification of the renal collecting systems. The ureters pass anteriorly to the transverse processes of the lumbar vertebrae. **(b)** Intravenous urogram, full-length view of the renal tract.

Relations of the right kidney

Superiorly and anteriorly: the right suprarenal gland and the liver. Anteriorly: the second part of the duodenum and the right colic flexure. Posteriorly: the diaphragm, costodiaphragmatic recess of the pleura, the 12th rib and muscles of the posterior abdominal wall.

Relations of the left kidney

Anteriorly: The left suprarenal gland, the spleen, the stomach, the pancreas, the left colic flexure, and loops of jejunum. Posteriorly: as for the right kidney.

Ureters

Anatomy of the ureters

Each ureter is a fibromuscular tube, lined with transitional mucosa, which is formed as the funnel of the renal pelvis narrows, at the pelvi-ureteric junction (PUJ) (Fig. 6.3). The ureters are approximately 1 cm in diameter and 25 cm long and run down the posterior abdominal wall inferiorly, along the psoas muscles (Fig. 6.3). At the pelvic brim, the ureters run anterior to the bifurcation of the common iliac vessels, in front of the sacro-iliac joint (Fig. 6.4). They then run down the posterolateral wall of the pelvis in close relation to the internal iliac vessels and, at the level of the ischial spines, turn anteromedially to join the trigone of the bladder at the vesico-ureteric junction (VUJ), which lies at the posterolateral angle of the bladder (Fig. 6.3). There are three normal narrowings of the ureters (where stones most commonly impact):

- at the pelvi-ureteric junction
- as the ureter crosses the pelvic brim
- at the vesico-ureteric junction.

Blood supply and lymphatic drainage of the ureters

The arterial supply to the upper ureter is from the ureteric branch of the renal artery. Branches of the gonadal artery supply the mid ureter. Branches of the internal iliac artery supply the lower ureter. There is accompanying venous drainage. Lymphatic drainage is into the lateral para-aortic nodes and the internal iliac nodes in the pelvis.

Nerve supply to the ureters

Sympathetic nerves to the ureters arise from the renal and gonadal plexuses (T12–L2) and, in the pelvis, from the hypogastric plexus. Afferent fibers return along the sympathetic pathways to enter the spinal canal at the L1 and L2 intervertebral foramina.

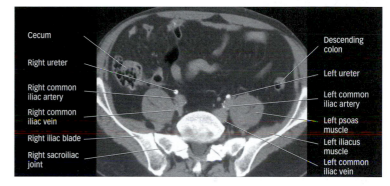

Fig. 6.4. **CT scan at the level of the pelvic brim, 10 minutes following intravenous contrast administration. At this time, contrast is seen within the ureters, which run down along the medial aspect of the psoas muscles, just anterior to the common iliac vessels.**

Relations of the ureters

Anteriorly (right): the duodenum (2nd part), the right gonadal, right colic and ileocolic vessels and the root of the small bowel mesentery, the terminal ileum and appendix. The right ureter lies lateral to the IVC.

Anteriorly (left): left gonadal and left colic vessels, loops of small and large bowel and the sigmoid mesocolon. The left ureter lies lateral to the aorta.

Posteriorly (right and left): the psoas muscles, and in the pelvis, the bifurcation of the left common iliac vessels. In the male pelvis, the ureter passes over the seminal vesicles and then hooks under the vas deferens before entering the bladder. In the female pelvis, the ureter runs inferior to the uterine artery in the broad ligament of the uterus, and lies adjacent to the lateral fornix of the vagina prior to entering the bladder.

Anatomical variants of the renal tract (Figs. 6.2(c), 6.5)

Several normal anatomical variants are seen which include:

- persistent fetal lobulation
- vascular anomalies (see above)
- renal duplication (the most common type of variant)
- incomplete or aberrant migration of the kidneys during embryogenesis.

Persistent fetal lobulation is a relatively common finding. Embryologically, each kidney arises from separate lobes that fuse together; in some cases, the lobulation remains visible (Fig. 6.5).

(a)

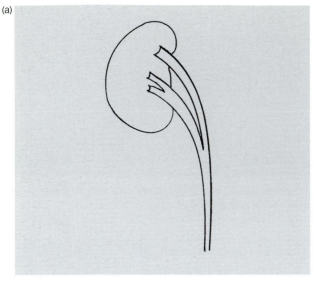

(b)

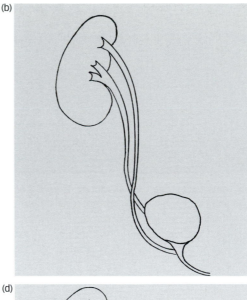

Fig. 6.5. **Anatomical variations of the kidney and ureters: (a) duplex kidney wth partial ureteric duplication, (b) duplex kidney, complete ureteric duplication and ectopic insertion of ureter from upper pole moiety into proximal ureter, (c) fetal lobulation, (d) cross-fused ectopia.**

(c)

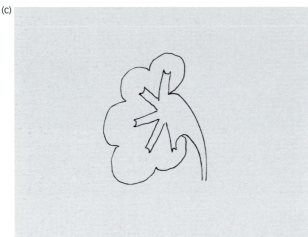

(d)

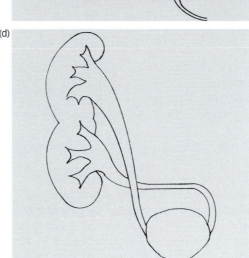

Renal duplication has an incidence of 2% and is bilateral in 20% of cases. In a classical duplex kidney, there are upper and lower pole moieties. Each moiety has a separate renal pelvis that drains into a separate ureter. The two ureters may join part of the way down between the kidney and bladder, forming a single distal ureter or, less commonly, may be duplicated throughout their length.

Abnormalities of migration occur less commonly. A pelvic kidney occurs in approximately 1 in 1500 deliveries. A horseshoe kidney (1 in 700 deliveries) occurs if there is fusion of the lower poles of both kidneys in the midline, with the upper poles lying on either side of the vertebral column. Crossed fused ectopia is where the lower pole of a normally sited kidney fuses with the upper pole of the contralateral kidney.

Imaging the kidneys and ureters
Ultrasound (Fig. 6.6) The renal cortex has a smooth border, may be slightly lobulated and is of intermediate echogenicity. The renal pyramids lie within the cortex and are relatively hypoechoic. The echogenic centre of the kidney consists of the renal pelvis surrounded by fat within the renal hilum. The renal pelvis and calyces are not usually seen unless they are distended due to distal obstruction, though the upper or lower parts of the ureter may be seen. The renal artery and vein are seen within the renal hilum.

Intravenous urogram (IVU) (Fig. 6.3) A plain film of the abdomen is first obtained to identify calcified renal tract stones. Iodinated contrast medium is then injected intravenously. The contrast medium is immediately concentrated in the renal tubules, resulting in a nephrogram, and progresses through the collecting tubules, draining into the renal calyces and pelvis. The cupped appearance of the calyces is well demonstrated (Fig. 6.3). The distribution of the major calyces to the upper, mid, and lower poles can be seen. Each major calyx drains through an infundibulum into the smooth funnel-shaped renal pelvis. The upper ureters form at the pelvi-ureteric junction and are depicted as smooth tubular structures running just medial to the tips of the transverse processes of the lumbar vertebrae, joining the bladder at the vesico-ureteric junction (see below).

CT may be performed without intravenous contrast (non-contrast CT). This technique is very sensitive in the identification of renal tract stones. The structure of the kidney is best demonstrated at the "cortico-medullary phase," which is at approximately 40 seconds following the intravenous administration of iodinated contrast medium (Fig. 6.2). The brightly enhancing renal cortex can be depicted clearly from the medulla at this phase. The central hilar fat is of low attenuation. The renal hilar vessels may be clearly depicted. On delayed imaging (at about 10 minutes), the kidney appears

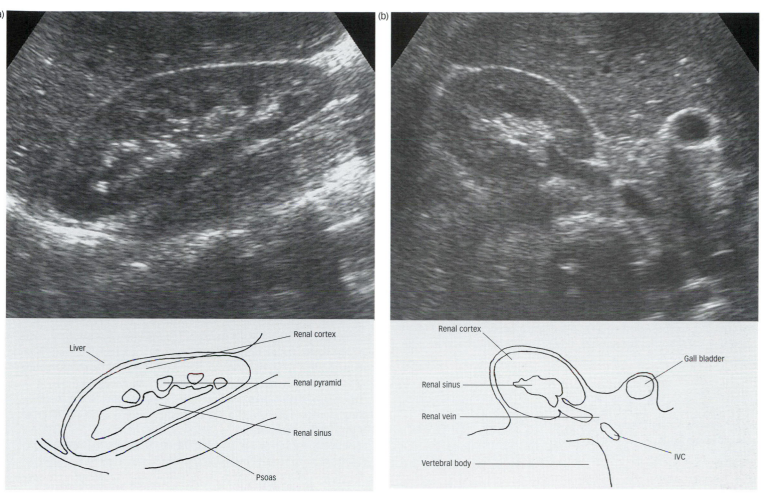

Fig. 6.6. **Ultrasound images showing the right kidney: (a) longitudinal and (b) axial.**

homogeneous and contrast may be seen in the renal pelvis and ureters down to the bladder (Fig. 6.4).

MRI (Fig. 6.1) The renal cortex and medulla are best depicted on T1 weighted images, where the cortex is intermediate and the medulla is low signal intensity. The renal pelvis and ureters are best depicted on T2 weighted images, where the urine within them appears of very high signal.

The anatomy of the renal vasculature may be depicted non-invasively following bolus contrast injection at CT and MRI. Early images demonstrate the arterial anatomy, which is then followed by the venous anatomy after a short delay (Fig. 6.2). Modern workstation software allows reformatting of the vessels in three dimensions.

Conventional angiography Since the advent of non-invasive CT and MR angiography, this invasive technique is reserved as the definitive test for demonstrating renal arterial anatomy and accessory vessels prior to a procedure such as stenting.

The suprarenal glands (Figs. 6.1, 6.7)
The right and left suprarenal glands (suprarenal glands) are endocrine glands, which lie anterior and superior to the medial aspect of the upper pole of the kidneys, at the level of T12. They are separated from

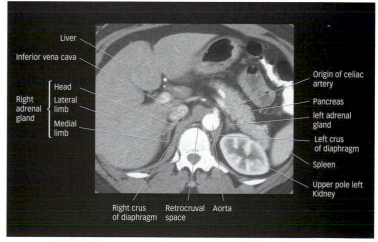

Fig. 6.7. **CT of the adrenal glands (arterial phase image). The adrenal glands are of soft tissue attenuation, surrounded by low attenuation fat.**

the kidneys by the perinephric fat, within Gerota's fascia. The glands consist of an outer cortex and an inner medulla.

The glands measure up to 5 cm in length and each limb measures between 2 mm and 6 mm transversely. The right adrenal gland usually has an "arrowhead" configuration. It lies posterior to the IVC, just above the upper pole of the right kidney. The left adrenal gland may have a pyramidal or crescentic configuration and lies along the antero-medial aspect of the left upper pole of kidney, between the upper pole and the renal hilum.

Blood supply and lymphatic drainage of the suprarenals

The arterial supply of the adrenals is from branches of the aorta, renal, and inferior phrenic arteries. A solitary vein drains directly into the IVC on the right and into the left renal vein on the left. Lymphatic drainage is to the lateral para-aortic nodes.

Nerve supply of the suprarenals

The nerve supply derives from the preganglionic sympathetic fibers of the splanchnic plexus. Preganglionic fibres from the splanchnic nerves also directly innervate cells of the adrenal medulla, to produce catecholamines.

Relations of the suprarenal glands

Right: The diagphragm lies posteriorly, with the right crus of diaphragm lying posteromedially. The upper pole of the right kidney lies inferolaterally and posteriorly. The IVC and right lobe of liver lie anteriorly.

Left: The diaphragm and left crus of diaphragm lie posteromedially. The upper pole of the left kidney lies posterolaterally. The peritoneum of the lesser sac, the stomach, the spleen, the splenic vein, and pancreas lie anteriorly.

Imaging the suprarenal glands

Ultrasound The suprarenal glands may be imaged in neonates when they are relatively large in relation to the kidneys. The glands gradually atrophy and are much more difficult to visualize on ultrasound in adults.

CT The glands are usually clearly seen as arrowhead or triangular soft tissue density structures, surrounded by the perinephric fat (Fig. 6.7). The glands are best depicted using fine sections through the gland (3–5 mm) following intravenous contrast medium. The limbs should be approximately the same width as the adjacent crus of diaphragm.

MRI (Fig. 6.1) The glands may be seen clearly on both axial and coronal images, particularly if surrounded by adequate perinephric fat.

The pelvic viscera
The bladder and urethra
The bladder

This is situated behind the pubic bones (Figs. 6.8 and 6.9). In the adult the empty bladder, which is pyramical in shape, lies entirely within the pelvis. The apex lies behind the upper border of the symphysis. The ureters enter the posterolateral angles of the triangular bladder base. The inferior angle or neck gives rise to the urethra, surrounded by the involuntary internal urethral sphincter. Posteriorly lies the vagina in the female and the vasa deferentia and seminal vesicles in the male. These structures are separated from the rectum by the rectovesical fascia. The superior surface of the bladder is completely covered by peritoneum. In the male, the neck of the bladder rests on the prostate gland, whereas in the female it rests directly on the pelvic fascia above the urogenital diaphragm. When the bladder fills, it becomes ovoid and the superior surface rises extraperitoneally into the abdomen.

Internally, the bladder wall is trabeculated except at the trigone, the triangular area between the two ureteric orifices superiorly and the urethral orifice inferiorly.

The blood supply to the bladder is from the superior and inferior vesical arteries. The veins of the vesical plexus drain to the internal iliac veins. Lymph drainage is to the internal iliac, thence to the para-aortic lymph nodes.

Imaging The bladder and ureters are opacified after intravenous urography (Fig. 6.3). In women, the fundus of the uterus indents the

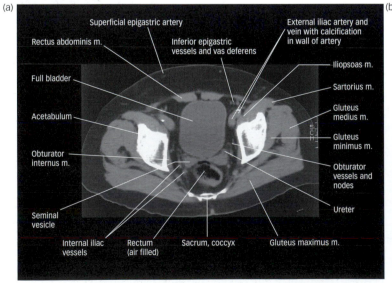
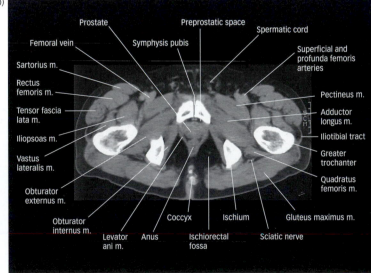

Fig. 6.8. **Axial CT of the male pelvis at the levels of (a) the acetabulum and (b) the symphysis pubis.**

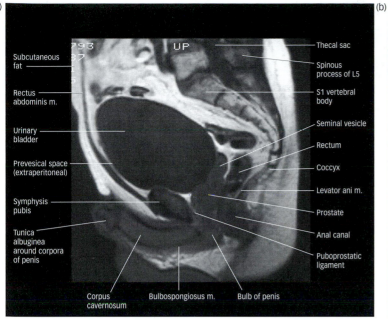

(a)

Subcutaneous fat

Rectus abdominis m.

Urinary bladder

Prevesical space (extraperitoneal)

Symphysis pubis

Tunica albuginea around corpora of penis

Thecal sac

Spinous process of L5

S1 vertebral body

Seminal vesicle

Rectum

Coccyx

Levator ani m.

Prostate

Anal canal

Puboprostatic ligament

Corpus cavernosum   Bulbospongiosus m.   Bulb of penis

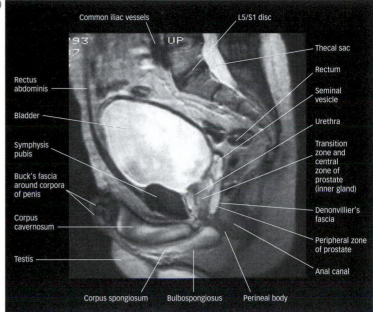

(b)

Common iliac vessels   L5/S1 disc

Rectus abdominis

Bladder

Symphysis pubis

Buck's fascia around corpora of penis

Corpus cavernosum

Testis

Thecal sac

Rectum

Seminal vesicle

Urethra

Transition zone and central zone of prostate (inner gland)

Denonvillier's fascia

Peripheral zone of prostate

Anal canal

Corpus spongiosum   Bulbospongiosus   Perineal body

Fig. 6.9. **Sagittal MR images of the male pelvis: (a) Tl weighted and (b) T2 weighted.**

dome of the bladder. In the male, the prostate gland may protrude up into the bladder base (the "prostatic impression"). The full bladder outline is smooth and regular, whereas after micturition, small amounts of contrast medium are seen trapped between the mucosal folds. The bladder can be filled with contrast retrogradely as part of a micturating cystourethrogram (MCUG).

On ultrasound of the full bladder, the echogenic wall should not exceed 4 mm in thickness (see Fig. 6.16). The bladder contents are trans-sonic. On CT, the bladder is best appreciated when filled with urine or contrast (Fig. 6.8). It has a rectangular shape and a wall thickness less than 4–5 mm. MR is ideal to demonstrate the relationships of the bladder in the coronal and sagittal planes (Figs. 6.9 and 6.10).

The male urethra

The male urethra is approximately 20 cm long and is divided into posterior (prostatic and membranous) and anterior (spongy) parts. The posterior urethra is 4 cm long and the anterior approximately 16 cm.

The prostatic urethra is 3 cm long. It is the widest part of the urethra. On its posterior wall is a ridge, the urethral or prostatic crest. In the middle of the crest is a further prominence, the verumontanum. On either side of this, the ejaculatory ducts (the common termination of the seminal vesicles and vasa deferentia) open.

The membranous urethra, 1.5 cm long, runs through the external urethral sphincter within the urogenital diaphragm. This is the narrowest, most fixed part of the urethra and is therefore most prone to injury.

The spongy urethra is further subdivided into the bulbous and penile urethra. It is surrounded by the corpus spongiosum. The long penile urethra is relatively narrow apart from a dilatation within the glans penis, the navicular fossa. The external urethral orifice is narrow and calculi may lodge at this site.

Imaging The urethra may be outlined with contrast medium retrogradely, with a balloon catheter in the navicular fossa. The anterior

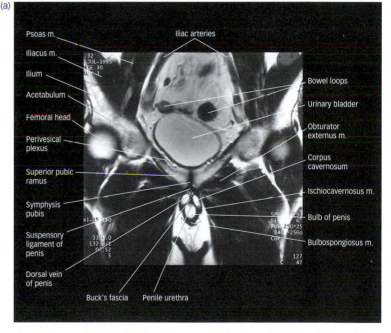

(a)

Psoas m.

Iliacus m.

Ilium

Acetabulum

Femoral head

Perivesical plexus

Superior pubic ramus

Symphysis pubis

Suspensory ligament of penis

Dorsal vein of penis

Iliac arteries

Bowel loops

Urinary bladder

Obturator externus m.

Corpus cavernosum

Ischiocavernosus m.

Bulb of penis

Bulbospongiosus m.

Buck's fascia   Penile urethra

Fig. 6.10. **Coronal T2 weighted MR images of the male pelvis: (a) to (c), from anterior to posterior. (Note chemical shift artifact from superior mid inferior bladder walls, anterior.)**

urethra is well visualized in this way, but demonstration of the posterior urethra may necessitate an MCUG (see above). It is also possible to image the anterior urethra with ultrasound.

The female urethra

This is 3–4 cm in length and extends from the neck of the bladder to the vestibule, where it opens 2.5 cm behind the clitoris. The female urethra may be visualized during MCUG.

(b)

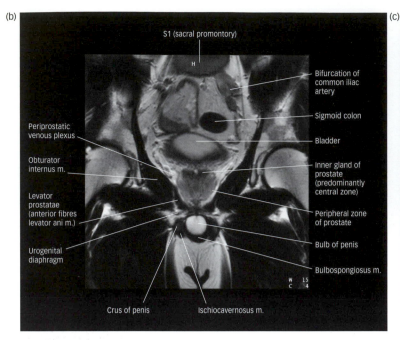

S1 (sacral promontory)

H

Periprostatic venous plexus

Obturator internus m.

Levator prostatae (anterior fibres levator ani m.)

Urogenital diaphragm

Crus of penis

Ischiocavernosus m.

Bifurcation of common iliac artery

Sigmoid colon

Bladder

Inner gland of prostate (predominantly central zone)

Peripheral zone of prostate

Bulb of penis

Bulbospongiosus m.

(c)

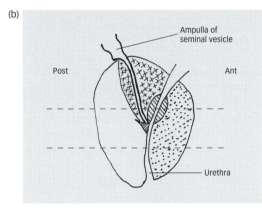

Median sacral artery

Ventral sacral foramen

H

Sacral plexus

Superior gluteal vessel

Periprostatic and perivesical venous plexus

Anal canal

Ischiorectal fossa

Sacroiliac joint

Gluteus medius

Sigmoid colon

Seminal vesicle

Obturator internus m.

Levator ani m.

Ischium

Quadratus femoris m.

Superficial transverse perineal m.

Fig. 6.10. *Continued*

(a)

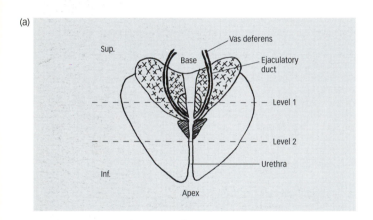

Sup.

Vas deferens

Base

Ejaculatory duct

Level 1

Level 2

Urethra

Inf.

Apex

(b)

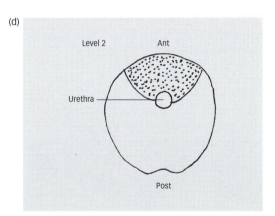

Ampulla of seminal vesicle

Post

Ant

Urethra

Fig. 6.11. **Diagrams of the zonal anatomy of the gland. (a) coronal; (b) sagittal; (c) and (d) axial at two different levels.**

▨ **Anterior fibromuscular stroma**
▧ **Central zone**
◨ **Transition zone**
▩ **Verumontanum**
☐ **Peripheral zone**

(c)

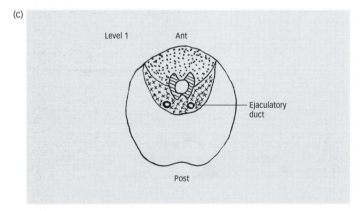

Level 1

Ant

Ejaculatory duct

Post

(d)

Level 2

Ant

Urethra

Post

The male genital tract
The prostate gland
The prostate gland is a pyramidal fibromuscular gland, 3.5 cm long, which surrounds the prostatic urethra from the bladder base to the urogenital diaphragm (Figs. 6.9, 6.10, and 6.11). The base, superiorly, is continuous with the bladder neck. The arch of the pubis lies

anteriorly. Laterally are the anterior fibers of the levator ani. Posteriorly lie the paired seminal vesicles. A fibrous sheath containing the periprostatic venous plexus surrounds it.

The ejaculatory ducts pierce the upper part of the posterior surface of the prostate and open into the prostatic urethra as described above.

The gland is divided into glandular and non-glandular tissue. The glandular tissue is subdivided into the peripheral zone or PZ (70%), the central zone or CZ (25%) and the transition zone or TZ (5%). The non-glandular fibromuscular stroma encircles the urethra anteriorly. Fig. 6.11 illustrates the zonal anatomy of the prostate diagrammatically.

The arterial supply to the prostate gland is from the inferior vesical and middle rectal arteries. Venous drainage is via the periprostatic plexus to the internal iliac veins and the vertebral venous plexus. Lymphatic drainage is to the internal iliac and obturator lymph nodes.

Imaging The prostate gland can be imaged by transabdominal ultrasound but transrectal ultrasound (TRUS) is superior (Fig. 6.12). The seminal vesicles are seen as hypoechoic sacculated structures postero-superior to the gland.

On CT, the prostate is seen as a rounded homogeneous soft tissue mass up to 3 cm in diameter.

On MRI, the gland is of uniformly low signal on T1W sequences, but T2W sequences demonstrate the zonal anatomy. The normal PZ has high signal intensity, as does the fluid within the seminal vesicles, whereas the CZ and TZ have relatively low signal. The term 'central gland' is often used to indicate the combined CZ and TZ. The anterior fibromuscular stroma is low signal on all sequences. Figures 6.8, 6.9, and 6.10 demonstrate the anatomy of the bladder and male genital tract in the sagittal, axial and coronal planes.

The seminal vesicles and ejaculatory ducts
The seminal vesicles are two lobulated sacs, about 5 cm long, which lie transversely behind the bladder and store semen. The terminal parts of the vasa deferentia lie medially. Posteriorly, the seminal vesicles are separated from the rectum by Denonvillier's fascia. Inferiorly, each seminal vesicle narrows and fuses with the ampulla of the vas deferens to form the ejaculatory ducts, each about 2 cm long.

Imaging On TRUS, the seminal vesicles appear as convoluted tubules, which contain transsonic fluid. They are less echogenic than the adjacent prostate. On CT, the seminal vesicles characteristically form a "bow tie" appearance in the groove between the bladder base and prostate (Fig. 6.8). On T2W MR sequences the fluid-containing seminal vesicles return a high signal (Fig. 6.10). The seminal vesicles are separated from the bladder by a high signal fat plane (Fig. 6.9).

The testis, epididymis, spermatic cord and vas deferens
The testes are ovoid reproductive and endocrine organs responsible for sperm production (Fig. 6.13). They lie within the scrotum, an out-pouching of the lower anterior abdominal wall, suspended by the spermatic cord. Each testis has an upper and lower pole and measures 4 cm by 2.5 cm by 3 cm. Each testis is surrounded by a tough fibrous capsule, the tunica albuginea, thickened posteriorly to form a fibrous septum, the mediastinum of the testis, in which the testicular vessels run. From here, fibrous septa divide the gland into 200–300 seminiferous lobules, each containing 1–3 seminiferous tubules. These drain to the mediastinum, from whence 10–15 efferent ducts pierce the tunica

(b)
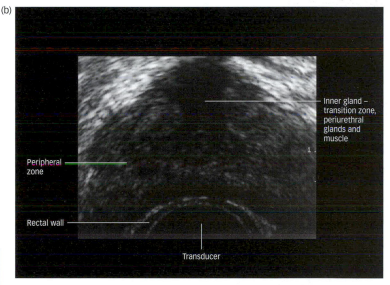

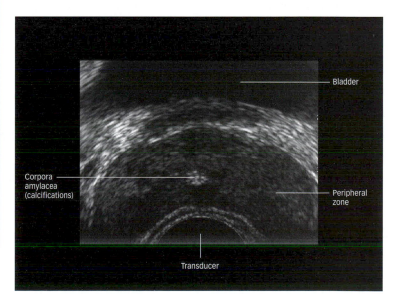

Fig. 6.12. **Transrectal ultrasound of the prostate gland: (a) longitudinal scan through the midline demonstrating the line of urethra, (b) transverse images of the prostate.**

(a)

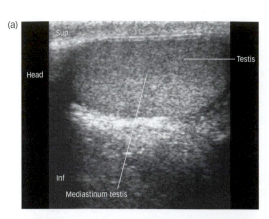

(b)

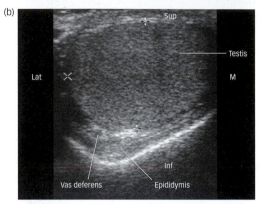

(c)

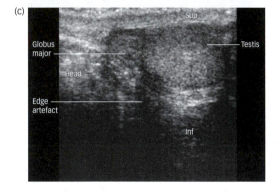

Fig. 6.13. **Ultrasound images of the testis: (a) longitudinal, (b) transverse and (c) longitudinal scans through the head of the epididymis (note typical streak artifact).**

The vas deferens is a muscular tube, 45 cm long, which conveys sperm to the ejaculatory ducts. The vas traverses the scrotum and spermatic cord to the deep inguinal ring, then runs back on the lateral pelvic wall to the ischial spine, where it turns medially to the bladder base, looping over the ureter. Its terminal dilatation, the ampulla, joins the seminal vesicle as described above.

Imaging At ultrasound, the testis has homogeneous medium level echoes throughout (Fig. 6.13). Coronal scans show the mediastinum as a line of high echogenicity posteriorly.

The epididymis is of similar, or slightly greater, echogenicity to the testis. The head of the epididymis, approximately 7–8 mm diameter, rests on the superior pole of the testis (Fig. 6.13).

The body and tail gradually decrease in thickness inferiorly to 1–2 mm. Duplex and color flow Doppler studies can demonstrate flow within the testicular arteries and veins.

At CT, the spermatic cord can be seen within the inguinal canal as a thin-walled, oval structure of fat attenuation containing small structures representing the vas and spermatic vessels (Fig. 6.8).

MR also provides excellent detail of the testis, having a homogeneous medium to low signal intensity on T1W images and high signal intensity on T2W images. The fibrous tunica albuginea is of low signal on all sequences. T2W images best depict the lower signal intensity of the mediastinum testis.

The penis

The root of the penis is described in the section on the perineum. The body of the penis comprises the two corpora cavernosa dorsally, separated by an incomplete fibrous septum, and the ventral corpus spongiosum surrounding the urethra. All three corpora are covered by a tough tube of fascia, the tunica albuginea, and Buck's fascia, continuous with the suspensory ligament of the penis, attached to the symphysis pubis. Distally, the corpus spongiosum expands to form the glans penis, which covers the distal corpora cavernosa. The arterial supply to the penis is from the dorsal artery, the artery to the bulb and the arteries to the crura. Venous drainage is mainly via the cavernous veins and the deep dorsal vein, which then drain to the internal pudendal veins. Lymphatic drainage from the body is to the superficial and deep inguinal nodes.

Imaging Ultrasound examination of the penis demonstrates low-level echoes within the corpora; the urethra is seen as a circular anechoic structure. Color flow and pulsed wave Doppler techniques allow visualization of the penile arteries, which is important in the assessment of erectile dysfunction. MRI may be used in the assessment of congental anomalies of the penis.

The female genital tract

The labia majora

The labia majora correspond to the scrotal sac of the male. The vestibular bulbs lie on either side of the vestibule into which the vagina and urethra open; they have erectile tissue and are covered by the bulbospongiosus muscles and the skin of the labia minora.

The vagina

The vagina is a muscular tube, approximately 8 cm long, which extends up and back from the vulva to surround the cervix of the uterus (Fig. 6.14). The vagina has anterior and posterior walls,

near the upper pole to enter the head of the epididymis. The efferent ducts fuse to form a single convoluted tube, which makes up the body and tail of the epididymis.

The epididymis lies posterolateral to the testis. It has a head superiorly, a body, and tail. Its overall length is 6–7 cm and it consists of the single convoluted duct. From the tail, the vas deferens ascends medially to the deep inguinal ring, within the spermatic cord.

The spermatic cord extends from the posterior border of the testis, on its medial side, to the deep inguinal ring. It contains the vas deferens, the testicular artery, and veins, the genital branch of the genitofemoral nerve and lymph vessels.

The testicular artery arises from the aorta at the level of the renal vessels. The scrotum is supplied by the external pudendal branch of the femoral artery. Venous drainage is via the pampiniform plexus of veins above and behind the testis, which becomes one single vein in the region of the inguinal ring. The testicular vein ascends to the IVC on the right and the renal vein on the left. Lymphatic drainage accompanies the testicular vessels to para-aortic lymph nodes at the level of Ll-2, whereas the scrotum drains to the superficial inguinal lymph nodes.

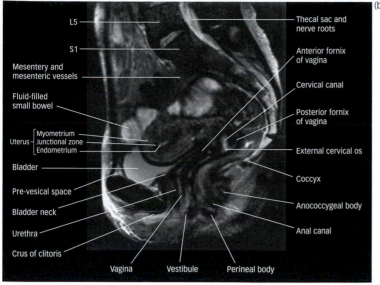

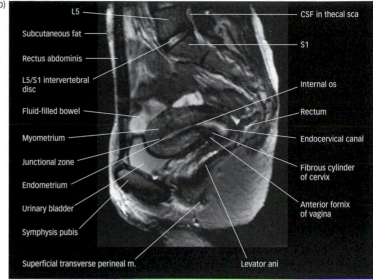

Fig. 6.14. **(a) Sagittal and (b) parasagittal T2 weighted images of the female pelvis, demonstrating the zonal anatomy of the uterus.**

normally in apposition. Superiorly, the cervix divides the vagina into shallow anterior and deep posterior and lateral fornices.

Anterior to the vagina are the bladder base and urethra. Posteriorly is the rectouterine pouch of Douglas and the ampulla of the rectum. The urethra, vagina, and rectum are all parallel to each other and to the pelvic brim.

Blood supply is via the vaginal artery and the vaginal branch of the uterine artery. The vaginal veins form a plexus that drains to the internal iliac veins. Lymphatic vessels from the upper two-thirds drain to the internal and external iliac nodes and from the lower third to the inguinal nodes.

Superiorly the vagina is supported by the levator ani, the transverse cervical (cardinal), pubocervical, and uterosacral ligaments, all attached to the vagina by pelvic fascia. Inferiorly, support is provided by the urogenital diaphragm and perineal body.

The uterus (Fig. 6.14 and 6.15)

The uterus is a pear-shaped muscular organ, approximately 8 cm long, 5 cm across and 3 cm thick. It has a fundus, body and cervix. The Fallopian tubes enter each superolateral angle (the cornu). The body narrows to a waist, the isthmus, below which lies the cervix, embraced by the vagina.

The cavity of the uterus is triangular in coronal section, but is a mere cleft in the sagittal plane. The cavity communicates with the cervical canal via the internal os, and the cervical canal opens into the vagina via the external os.

Peritoneum covers the entire uterus except below the level of the internal os anteriorly, where it is reflected on to the bladder, and laterally between the layers of the broad ligament. The thick smooth muscle myometrium is related directly to the endometrium with no intervening submucosa. The endometrium is continuous with the mucous membrane of the uterine tubes and the endocervix.

The main arterial supply of the uterus is the uterine artery, which passes to the uterus in the base of the broad ligament, crossing above the ureter. The artery anastomoses with the ovarian artery. The vein

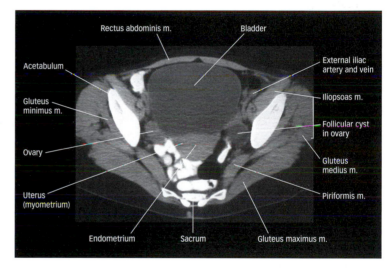

Fig. 6.15. **Axial CT of the female pelvis at a level above the acetabulum to show the normal uterus and ovaries.**

accompanies the artery and drains into the internal iliac vein. Lymphatic vessels drain to internal and external iliac lymph nodes and para-aortic nodes.

Uterine ligaments and supports include: (a) the levator ani muscles; (b) the transverse cervical, pubocervical, and uterosacral ligaments, (c) the broad and round ligaments.

The broad ligaments are formed by anterior and posterior reflections of peritoneum passing over the Fallopian tubes. They enclose the parametrial connective tissue in addition to the round ligaments, uterine vessels, and accompanying lymph channels and ovarian ligaments laterally.

The uterine tubes

Each Fallopian tube is about 10 cm long and lies in the free edge of the broad ligament, extending out from the uterine cornua to form a funnel-shaped lateral part, the infundibulum, which extends beyond the broad ligament and overhangs the ovary with its finger-like fimbriae.

Arterial supply is from the ovarian and uterine arteries and there is corresponding venous drainage. Lymphatic drainage is chiefly to para-aortic lymph nodes.

The ovaries

These paired almond-shaped reproductive and endocrine organs lie in the ovarian f'ossae, situated in the lateral pelvic sidewalls. Their size and appearance varies with age. Normal adult dimensions are 3 × 1.5 × 2 cm with a weight of 2–8 g and each ovary contains a few mature follicles, 70 000 immature follicles, and postovulatory corpora lutea and corpora albicantia (scarred areas marking the site of previously ruptured follicles). After the menopause, the ovary atrophies.

The ovary is attached to the back of the broad ligament by the mesovarium. It is attached to the infundibulum of the Fallopian tube as described above. That part of the broad ligament lateral to the mesovarium running to the lateral pelvic wall is known as the suspensory ligament of the ovary and within it run the ovarian vessels and lymphatics. Inferiorly lies the levator ani muscle.

Arterial supply is by the ovarian artery, which arises from the aorta at Ll/2. Venous drainage is from the pampiniform plexus into the ovarian veins, which drain into the IVC on the right and the renal vein on the left. Lymph drainage is along the ovarian vessels to preaortic lymph nodes at the level of the first and second lumbar vertebra.

Imaging The commonest method of investigation of the female genital tract is with ultrasound. The full urinary bladder provides an acoustic window through which the uterus and ovaries may be visualized. In the adult the myometrium is of uniform low echogenicity and the endometrium is seen as a highly echogenic stripe on longitudinal images. The thickness of the central echogenic stripe depends on the phase of the menstrual cycle, being maximal perimenstrually (Fig. 6.16). Postmenopausally, the thickness and echogenicity of the endometrium is reduced.

The vagina is seen inferiorly on sagittal scans as a highly echogenic stripe making an acute angle with the body of the uterus. The ovaries can usually be identified in the adnexal areas and in the adult it is possible to see up to five or six small transsonic follicles. It is normal to see a small amount of fluid in the pouch of Douglas. Endovaginal ultrasound provides much improved resolution (Fig. 6.17). It is possible to demonstrate the vascular supply of the ovaries with color Doppler. Ultrasound is capable of demonstrating most congenital abnormalities of the uterus.

On CT scans, the uterus is seen as a homogeneous soft tissue mass dorsal to the bladder (Fig. 6.15), but it is not usually possible to recognize the ovaries unless they are enlarged or contain cysts. The broad ligament appears as a thin, soft tissue density extending anterolaterally from the uterus to the pelvic sidewalls.

On T2W MRI sequences in the adult (Fig. 6.14), three distinct zones are seen within the uterus: the endometrium, junctional zone (JZ), and myometrium. The endometrium and uterine cavity appear as a high signal stripe, bordered by the low signal intensity JZ. This represents the inner myometrium and, at the level of the internal os, it blends with the low signal band of fibrous cervical stroma. The outer

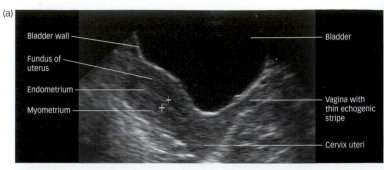

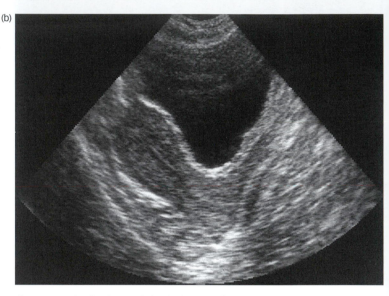

Fig. 6.16. **Longitudinal transabdominal scans of the uterus: (a) secretory phase, (b) proliferative phase. Note the difference in thickness of endometrium.**

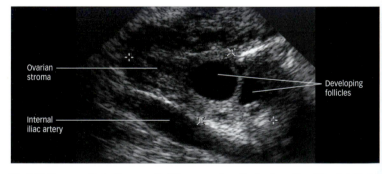

Fig. 6.17. **Transvaginal ultrasound of the ovary, longitudinal section. The detailed structure of the ovary and follicles can be visualized.**

myometrium is of intermediate signal intensity, which increases in the midsecretory phase.

On T2W images the cervix has an inner cylinder of low signal stroma continuous with the JZ. The appearances do not change with the menstrual cycle or with oral contraceptives.

Normal ovaries are low to medium signal on T1W images and higher signal on T2W images. Follicles stand out as round hyperintense foci.

The anatomy of the Fallopian tubes and fine mucosal detail of the uterine cavity are best demonstrated by hysterosalpingography (HSG)

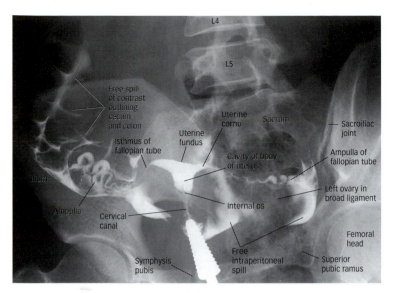

Fig. 6.18. **Normal hysterosalpingogram (HSG).**

(Fig. 6.18). The uterine cavity is usually triangular and smooth walled, leading to the narrow Fallopian tubes. Contrast should spill freely into the peritoneal cavity.

The posterior abdominal wall
Bones and muscles of the posterior abdominal wall
The five lumbar vertebrae run down the midline of the posterior abdominal wall, separated by the intervertebral discs. The 12th rib forms the superior margin of the posterior abdominal wall.

Muscles and fascia (Fig. 6.19)
Psoas The paired psoas muscles arise from the roots of the transverse processes, the vertebral bodies and intervertebral discs of the 12th thoracic to 5th lumbar vertebrae (Fig. 6.1 and 6.2). Each is enclosed in a fibrous sheath derived from the lumbar fascia, which covers the internal layer of the posterior abdominal wall musculature. Each psoas muscle runs inferolaterally, where it is joined by the fibers of iliacus to form the iliopsoas muscle, passing behind the inguinal ligament to insert into the lesser trochanter of the femur (Fig. 6.8). The nerve supply is from the lumbar plexus.

Iliacus This paired fan-shaped muscle arises from the upper part of the iliac fossa. The fibres join the lateral side of psoas tendon as described above.

Quadratus lumborum This paired flat muscle arises below from the iliolumbar ligament, adjoining iliac crest and the tips of the transverse processes of the lower lumbar vertebrae (Fig. 6.2). Fibers run superiorly and medially to insert into the lower border of the 12th rib. The anterior surface is covered by the lumbar fascia. The nerve supply is via the lumbar plexus.

Transversus abdominis This is the deepest of the three sheets of muscle that form the anterior abdominal wall. Near the lateral border of quadratus lumborum, the muscle becomes a fibrous aponeurotic sheet that splits into two layers to surround the muscles of the posterior abdominal wall, forming the anterior and posterior parts of the thoracolumbar fascia.

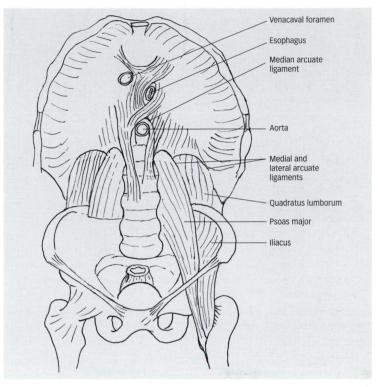

Fig. 6.19. **The muscles of the posterior abdominal wall.**

Diaphragm This is formed by a peripheral muscular component and a central tendinous component.

The muscular part of the diaphragm is composed of:

* vertebral component (the crura and the medial and lateral arcuate ligaments)
* costal component, which attaches to the inferior costal margin
* sternal component, which attaches to the xiphisternum.

The crura insert onto the anterior vertebral bodies from L1 to L3 on the right and L1 to L2 on the left. The crura join in the midline to form a tendon, the median arcuate ligament. The medial and lateral arcuate ligaments are the fascial thickenings over the psoas and quadratus lumborum muscles, giving origin to the diaphragm.

The central tendinous part of the diaphragm is fused with the pericardium. It is pierced by the IVC (at T8). The aorta passes through the diaphragm posterior to the median arcuate ligament, in the retro-crural space (at T12). The esophagus passes through th muscular part of the diaphragm in the region of the right crus (at T10).

Muscles of the pelvis
The major muscles include the paired psoas and iliacus muscles, described above. Within the true pelvis, the piriformis muscles, covered by parietal fascia, arise on either side of the anterior sacrum and pass laterally through the greater sciatic foramen to insert onto the greater trochanter of the femur, so forming part of the posterior wall of the pelvis (see Fig. 6.15).

The lateral wall of the pelvis is formed by the obturator internus muscle, covering the tough obturator membrane, which overlies the obturator foramen (Fig. 6.10). A small deficiency anteriorly forms the obturator canal, through which the obturator vessels and nerve pass to

(a)

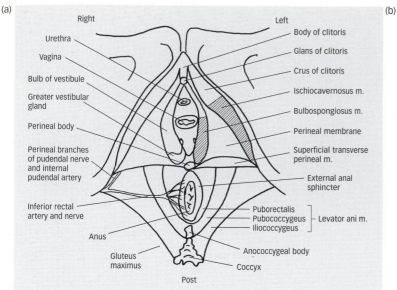

(b)

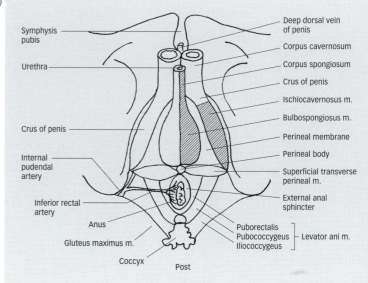

Fig. 6.20. **Diagrams of (a) the female and (b) male peritoneum, viewed from below. The cross-hatching indicates the muscles overlying the crura and bulb of the clitoris and vestibule (female) and the penis (male).**

enter the thigh. The tendon of obturator internus runs through the lesser sciatic foramen to insert onto the lesser trochanter of the femur.

The pelvic floor

MR, with its multiplanar capability, is particularly well suited to demonstration of the pelvic floor (Figs. 6.10 and 6.14). On T1-weighted sequences (T1W) the high signal pelvic fat provides excellent contrast with the low signal pelvic musculature.

The pelvic floor supports the pelvic viscera and is composed of a funnel-shaped sling of muscles and fascia pierced by the rectum, the urethra and, in the female, the vagina. The muscle groups are divided into:

(a) the pelvic diaphragm superiorly: levator ani and coccygeus
(b) the perineal muscles inferiorly (Fig. 6.20): the urogenital perineum anteriorly and the anal perineum posteriorly.

The levator ani is the most important muscle of the pelvic floor. It arises from the posterior aspect of the pubis, the pelvic fascia over obturator internus and the ischial spine.

The levatores ani act as a muscular support and have a sphincter action on the anorectal junction and vagina. They are assisted by the small coccygeus muscles posteriorly (Fig. 6.20).

The perineum is a diamond-shaped space that lies within the ischiopubic rami and the coccyx. A line drawn between the ischial tuberosities will pass just anterior to the anus, demarcating the urogenital triangle anteriorly and the anal triangle posteriorly (Fig. 6.20).

The anterior urogenital triangle contains the musculofascial urogenital diaphragm, which is pierced by the urethra in both sexes, forming the voluntary sphincter urethrae, and by the vagina in the female. Below this is the superficial perineal pouch, which in the male contains: (a) the bulbospongiosus muscle which covers the corpus spongiosum and surrounds the urethra, the whole forming the bulb of the penis; (b) the paired ischiocavernosus muscles which arise from the ischial ramus and cover the corpora cavernosa of the penis (Fig. 6.20).

The same muscles are present in the female although they are less well developed (Fig. 6.20). In the midline, at the junction of the anterior and posterior perineum, lies the fibromuscular perineal body, to which the anal sphincter and perineal muscles attach (Fig. 6.20).

The anal triangle, between the ischial tuberosities and coccyx, contains the anus and its sphincters, levator ani and, laterally, the ischiorectal fossae (figure 10). These lie below and lateral to the posterior fibres of levator ani.

The blood and lymph supply to the abdomen and pelvis
The abdominal aorta

The abdominal aorta is a continuation of the thoracic aorta as it passes through the diaphragmatic hiatus, just anterior to the 12th thoracic vertebra (Figs. 6.1 and 6.2), accompanied by the thoracic duct, azygous and hemi-azygous veins splanchnic nerves and sympathetic trunks. The diaphragmatic crura envelope the anterolateral aspect of the aorta and then insert into the 1st or 2nd lumbar levels (Fig. 6.7).

The aorta runs along the anterior aspect of the lumbar vertebrae, slightly to the left of the midline, down to the 4th lumbar vertebra, where its terminal divisions are the common iliac arteries and the median sacral artery. The IVC, the cysterna chyli and the origin of the azygous vein lie to the right of the aorta. The sympathetic trunk runs closely applied to the left side of the aorta.

Many of the branches of the aorta may be demonstrated with ultrasound (Fig. 6.21) and angiography (including CT, MR angiography and direct angiography) (Fig. 6.22):

The branches of the aorta include:
Three anterior arteries:

- celiac artery (at T12/L1), dividing into the hepatic artery and splenic arteries, supplying the liver, stomach, pancreas, and spleen
- superior mesenteric artery (at L1), dividing into the inferior pancreaticoduodenal artery, the jejunal and ileal arteries, the middle colic, right colic, and ileocolic arteries, supplying the mid-gut, to the mid-transverse colon

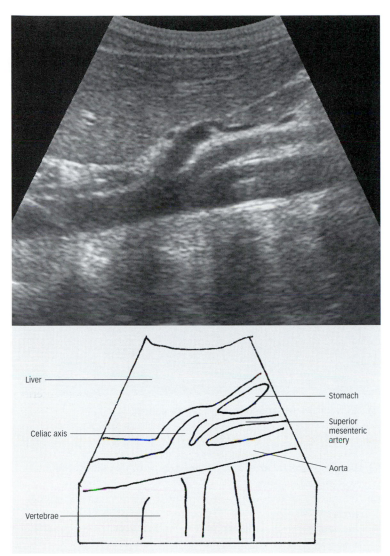

Fig. 6.21. **Longitudinal ultrasound scan through the aorta, celiac, and superior mesenteric arteries.**

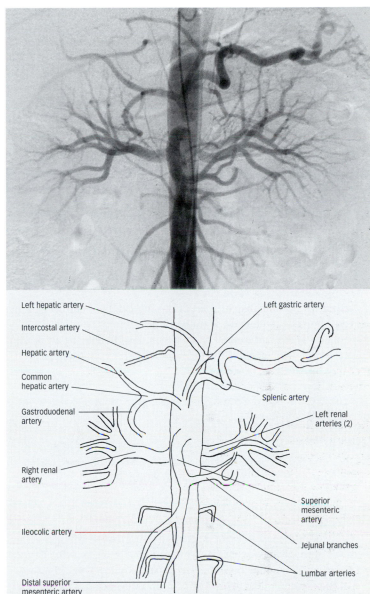

Fig. 6.22. **Flush aortogram, frontal projection. Note the left hepatic artery arises from the left gastric artery (a variant seen in 25% of normal individuals). The patient has two left renal arteries.**

- inferior mesenteric artery (at L3), dividing into the superior left colic artery, inferior left colic arteries, and the superior rectal artery.

Three pairs of lateral visceral arteries:

- adrenal arteries
- renal arteries
- gonadal arteries (testicular or ovarian).

Five pairs of lateral abdominal wall arteries:

- inferior phrenic arteries (supplying the diaphragm)
- four pairs of lumbar arteries (supplying the abdominal wall).

Imaging the aorta

Ultrasound: The abdominal aorta may be imaged from the diaphragm to the bifurcation, although occasionally the distal aorta is obscured by overlying bowel gas. It is normally 2–3 cm in diameter (Fig. 6.21).

CT and MRI: The aorta and its main branches are well depicted on CT and MRI following intravenous contrast enhancement (Figs. 6.1, 6.2 and 6.7). The celiac axis, superior mesenteric artery and renal arteries are always visible when normal. The inferior mesenteric artery and several lumbar arteries may also be seen. Multi-detector CT or MR angiography enable image reformatting, to demonstrate the vessels in any anatomical plane.

Angiography: A pigtail catheter introduced into the upper abdominal aorta is used to inject iodinated contrast medium directly into the aorta, followed by rapid imaging (Fig. 6.22). Selective catheterization of the aortic branches may also be performed.

Inferior vena cava (IVC) (Figs. 6.2, 6.7)

The IVC is formed by the union of the common iliac veins from the pelvis, just behind the right common iliac artery, at the level of the 4th or 5th lumbar vertebra. The IVC runs up along the anterior aspects of the lumbar vertebral bodies, just to the right of the aorta. It runs anterior to the right adrenal gland and right crus of diaphragm. Superiorly, the IVC runs through the liver (the intrahepatic IVC). It then crosses through the central tendon of the diaphragm at the level of the 8th thoracic vertebra to drain into the right atrium of the heart.

Tributaries that drain into the IVC closely follow the branches of the aorta (apart from the venous drainage of the small and large bowel, which is via the mesenteric veins that drain into the portal circulation):

- abdominal wall veins drain into the IVC via the right and left phrenic veins and the 3rd and 4th lumbar veins
- the right gonadal, renal and adrenal veins each drain directly into the IVC
- the left gonadal and adrenal veins drain into the left renal vein, which then crosses the midline and drains into the IVC
- the right, middle and left hepatic veins drain into the intrahepatic IVC.

Imaging the inferior vena cava

Ultrasound: The intrahepatic part of the IVC can be seen throughout its length, up to the junction with the right atrium. The upper abdominal portion of IVC can usually be well seen, but the lower part of the IVC, common iliac, internal and external iliac veins are often partly obscured by overlying bowel gas.

CT: The IVC can be seen throughout its length. The major pelvic veins are also well demonstrated.

MRI: This is the method of choice for the demonstration of flow in the IVC. The images are best performed as an MR venogram, with administration of intravenous contrast medium (Fig. 6.2).

The pelvic vasculature

A pelvic arteriogram is shown in Fig. 6.23.

The aorta bifurcates in front of the fourth lumbar vertebral body at the level of the iliac crest into the common iliac arteries, which enter the pelvis on the medial border of the psoas muscles, lying just anterior to the common iliac veins. The common iliac arteries divide at the pelvic brim anterior to the lower sacroiliac joints into internal and external iliac arteries.

The external iliac artery runs along the medial border of psoas, passing under the inguinal ligament to become the femoral artery. It is larger than the internal iliac artery. Just above the inguinal ligament, it gives off the inferior epigastric artery and the deep circumflex iliac artery, which supply the anterior abdominal wall muscles.

The internal iliac artery enters the true pelvis anterior to the sacroiliac joint, with the ureter anterior to it. From its origin, the artery runs inferomedially, anterior to the sacrum, its length varying from 2–5 cm. It has the most variable branching pattern of all the arteries in the body; the commonest pattern is described here. It divides into anterior and posterior divisions at the upper border of the greater sciatic foramen.

The anterior division courses down towards the ischial spine and gives off the following branches:

(a) the obturator artery
(b) the inferior vesical artery, supplying the lower bladder, ureter, prostate gland and seminal vesicles

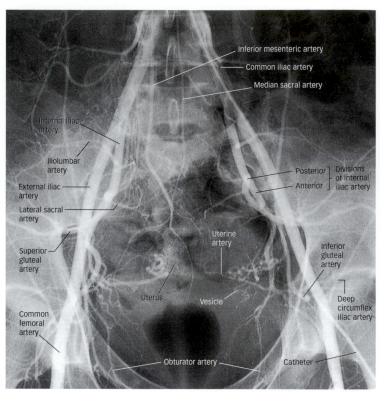

Fig. 6.23. **Normal pelvic arteriogram in a female patient.**

(c) the middle rectal artery, supplying the prostate gland, seminal vesicles and rectum
(d) the uterine artery, supplying the uterus, upper vagina, Fallopian tubes and ovary
(e) the vaginal artery, equivalent to the inferior vesical artery in the male
(f) the internal pudendal artery, supplying the genitalia in the perineum
(g) the superior vesical artery, supplying the upper bladder
(h) the inferior gluteal artery, which passes through the lower part of the greater sciatic foramen.

Branches of the posterior division of the internal iliac artery are as follows:

(a) the iliolumbar artery, supplying psoas and iliacus
(b) the lateral sacral artery, which supplies the sacral canal and the muscles and skin over the back
(c) the superior gluteal artery, the largest branch of the internal iliac artery, passing through the greater sciatic foramen to the gluteal region.

The internal and external iliac veins accompany the arteries. MR and CT can demonstrate the pelvic vasculature.

Lymphatics of the abdomen and pelvis

Lymph nodes and lymphatic vessels accompany the major vessels of the abdomen and pelvis and are classified accordingly. In the pelvis, the internal and external iliac lymph nodes drain to common iliac lymph nodes and thence to para-aortic lymph nodes (see below).

Pre-aortic nodes are clustered around the origins of the celiac axis, the superior mesenteric artery and the inferior mesenteric artery. These drain the gastrointestinal tract from the lower esophagus to half-way down the anal canal, as well as the spleen, pancreas, gall bladder, and part of the liver.

The left para-aortic nodes are grouped along the left lateral aspect of the aorta. The right para-aortic nodes lie anterior and lateral to the IVC. The para-aortic nodes drain lymph from the kidneys and adrenal glands, from the testes in the male and the ovaries, Fallopian tubes and uterine fundus in the female. The para-aortic nodes drain into two lymph vessels, the right and left lumbar trunks. The right and left lumbar trunks join the intestinal trunk to form the cisterna chyli. This lies just to the right of the aorta, behind the right crus of diaphragm, at the level of L1/L2 and is approximately 6 cm long. The cisterna chyli then drains into the thoracic duct (see chapter "Thorax" section titled "thoracic duct").

Imaging the abdominal lymphatic system

Ultrasound: Although the para-aortic lymph nodes in the upper abdomen may be seen in thin patients, lymph node assessment is usually incomplete because of overlying bowel gas.

CT and MRI: Lymph nodes can be seen when they measure approximately 3 mm or more in short axis diameter. Normal para-aortic nodes may measure up to 1 cm in short axis diameter. Pelvic lymph nodes rarely exceed 8 mm in short axis diameter.

Lumbosacral plexus

The lumbar plexus is formed in the psoas muscle from the anterior rami of the L1 to L4 nerve roots. The nerves that form include:

- the iliohypogastric and ilioinguinal nerves
- the lateral cutaneous nerve of the thigh
- the femoral nerve (L 2,3,4), which may be visualized as it runs down and laterally between the psoas and iliacus to enter the thigh beneath the inguinal ligament
- the genitofemoral nerve
- the obturator nerve (L2, 3, 4), which crosses the pelvic brim anterior to the sacroiliac joint, runs behind the common iliac vessels, and down the pelvic side-wall into the obturator canal (Fig. 6.8)
- the L4 root of the lumbosacral trunk, which joins sacral roots in the sacral plexus.

The sacral plexus, formed from the lumbosacral trunk (L4, 5) and the ventral rami of the first to fourth sacral nerves, lies on the piriformis muscle (Fig. 6.10c). The largest branch is the sciatic nerve, which may be visualized by CT and MR as it passes through the greater sciatic foramen into the gluteal region (Fig. 6.8b).

Abdominal sympathetic trunk and sympathetic plexus

The abdominal sympathetic trunks enter the abdomen through the medial arcuate ligaments as continuations of the thoracic sympathetic trunks and run along the anterior lumbar vertebrae, then continue as the pelvic sympathetic chains in the pelvis, posterior to the common iliac vessels. They are not usually seen using current imaging techniques.

PAUL BUTLER

Anatomical Overview

The brain is supported by the skull base and enclosed within the skull vault. Within, the cranial cavity is divided into the anterior, middle and posterior fossae. The anterior and middle cranial fossae contain the two cerebral hemispheres. The posterior fossa contains the brainstem, consisting of the midbrain, pons and, most inferiorly, the medulla, and the cerebellum. Twelve paired cranial nerves arise from the brainstem, exit the skull base through a number of foramina, and innervate a variety of structures in the head proper. The largest of these foramina is the foramen magnum, through which the brainstem and spinal cord are in continuity. The brain is invested by the meninges and bathed in cerebrospinal fluid (CSF), circulating in the subarachnoid space. Part of the meninges, the dura, forms an incomplete partition between the cerebral hemispheres, known as the falx and roofs the posterior fossa as the tentorium cerebelli. There is a gap in the tentorium, called the hiatus, through which the midbrain joins the hemispheres.

Within the brain are a number of cavities, the lateral, third and fourth cerebral ventricles, which contain CSF produced by the choroid plexuses within the ventricles. CSF flows from the ventricles into the subarachnoid spaces over the cerebral surface and around the spinal cord.

Blood reaches the brain by the carotid and vertebral arteries and is drained by cerebral veins into a series of sinuses within the dura into the internal jugular veins.

Imaging overview

CT and MRI scanning are central to neuroimaging. The role of skull radiography is very limited and arguably the only situation where it enjoys a primary role is in the investigation of skull fractures in suspected non-accidental injury in children. The relative merits of MRI and CT in are summarized below and routine series of axial MRI and CT are illustrated in Figs. 7.1 and 7.2.

(a)

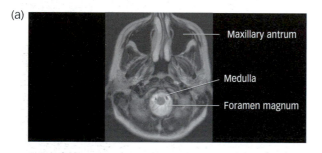

Maxillary antrum

Medulla

Foramen magnum

(b)

Vertebral artery

Medulla

(c)

basilar artery

hypoglossal nerve canal

foramen of Luschka

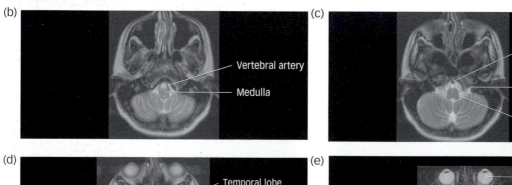

(d)

Temporal lobe

Meckel's cave

Middle cerebellar peduncle

Inferior cerebellar peduncle

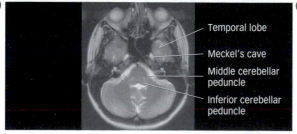

(e)

Globe
Lateral rectus
Sphenoid sinus
Internal carotid artery
Trigeminal nerve

Pons

Middle cerebellar peduncle

Fourth ventricle

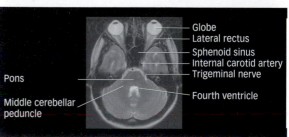

Fig. 7.1.

Routine T2 weighted axial cranial MRI: (a) to (o), base to vertex.

Applied Radiological Anatomy for Medical Students. Paul Butler, Adam Mitchell, and Harold Ellis (eds.) Published by Cambridge University Press. © P. Butler, A. Mitchell, and H. Ellis 2007.

Fig. 7.1.
Continued

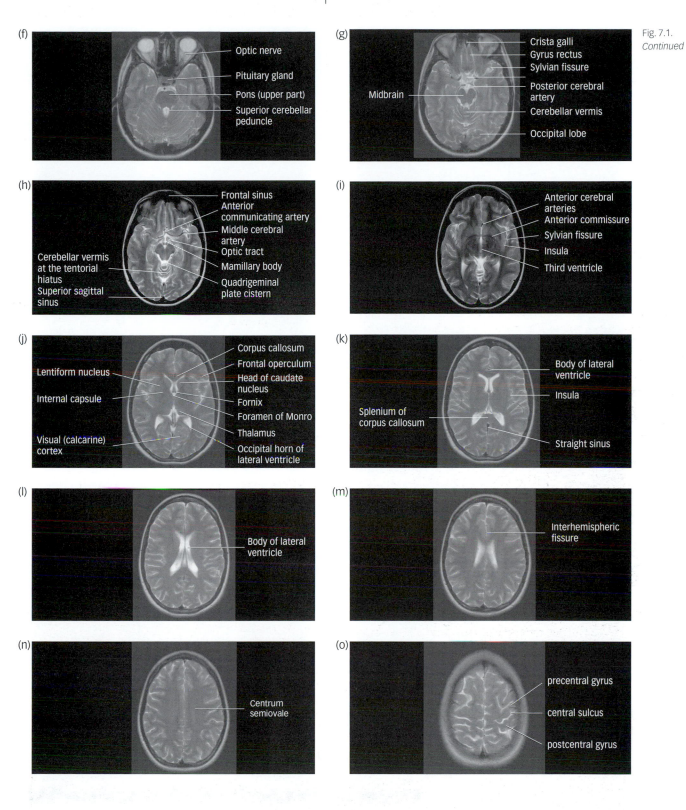

(f)
Optic nerve
Pituitary gland
Pons (upper part)
Superior cerebellar peduncle

(g)
Crista galli
Gyrus rectus
Sylvian fissure
Posterior cerebral artery
Midbrain
Cerebellar vermis
Occipital lobe

(h)
Frontal sinus
Anterior communicating artery
Middle cerebral artery
Optic tract
Mamillary body
Quadrigeminal plate cistern
Cerebellar vermis at the tentorial hiatus
Superior sagittal sinus

(i)
Anterior cerebral arteries
Anterior commissure
Sylvian fissure
Insula
Third ventricle

(j)
Corpus callosum
Frontal operculum
Head of caudate nucleus
Fornix
Foramen of Monro
Thalamus
Occipital horn of lateral ventricle
Lentiform nucleus
Internal capsule
Visual (calcarine) cortex

(k)
Body of lateral ventricle
Insula
Splenium of corpus callosum
Straight sinus

(l)
Body of lateral ventricle

(m)
Interhemispheric fissure

(n)
Centrum semiovale

(o)
precentral gyrus
central sulcus
postcentral gyrus

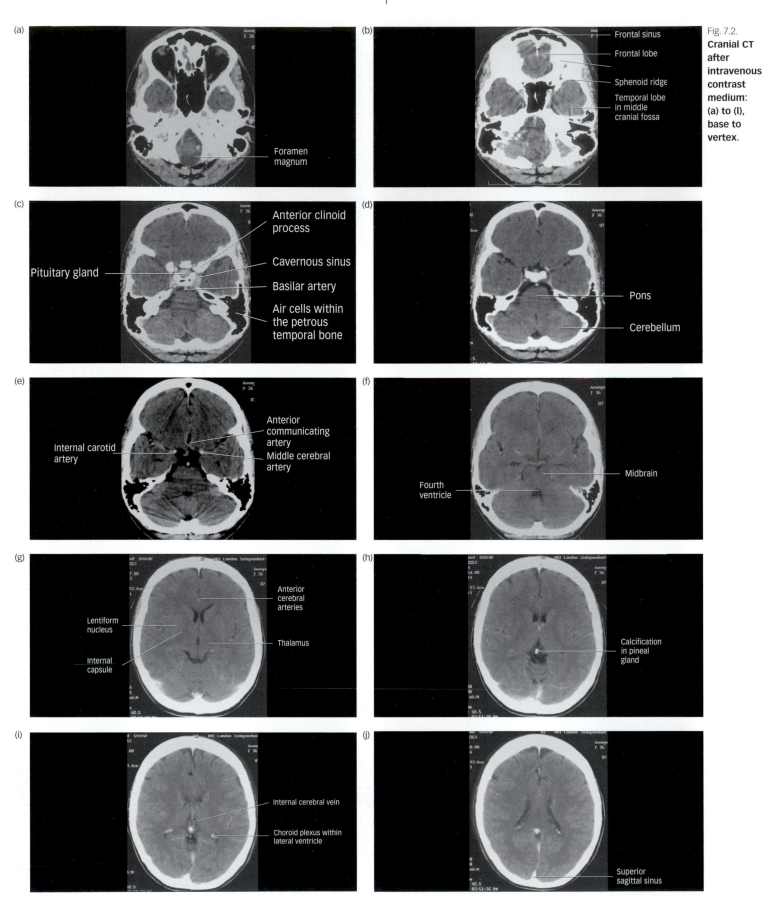

(a) Foramen magnum

(b) Frontal sinus
Frontal lobe
Sphenoid ridge
Temporal lobe in middle cranial fossa

Fig. 7.2.
Cranial CT after intravenous contrast medium: (a) to (l), base to vertex.

(c) Anterior clinoid process
Cavernous sinus
Basilar artery
Air cells within the petrous temporal bone
Pituitary gland

(d) Pons
Cerebellum

(e) Anterior communicating artery
Middle cerebral artery
Internal carotid artery

(f) Midbrain
Fourth ventricle

(g) Anterior cerebral arteries
Thalamus
Lentiform nucleus
Internal capsule

(h) Calcification in pineal gland

(i) Internal cerebral vein
Choroid plexus within lateral ventricle

(j) Superior sagittal sinus

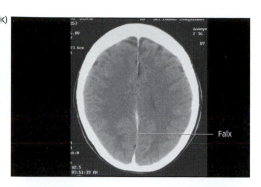

Fig. 7.2. *Continued*

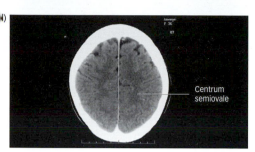

MRI
Advantages

- Superior anatomical detail
- Superior contrast resolution
- Multiplanar capability
- Better for middle and posterior cranial fossae
- No ionizing radiation.

Disadvantages

- Longer investigation
- Claustrophobia
- A number of contraindications relating to various metallic implants (surgical clips, pacemakers, etc.) and the use of high field-strength magnets
- Insensitive to subarachnoid haemorrhage and calcification.

CT
Advantages

- Excellent for the emergency situation, both traumatic and non-traumatic.
- Quick and simple for the patient
- Good for hemorrhage and calcification.

Disadvantages

- Ionizing radiation
- Streak artifacts from bone limit visualization of the adjacent structures (e.g., the contents of the middle and posterior fossae).
- Usually restricted to axial images with the patient supine, although high quality, multiplanar views can be reconstructed on the modern scanners.

MRI is concerned with proton (hydrogen nucleus) imaging and different images can be produced depending on the parameters used (the different pulse sequences). On the T1 weighted (T1W), images, gray matter is darker (lower signal intensity) than white matter. On T2 weighted (T2W), sequences, the reverse is true. Broadly, T1W images are good for anatomy, T2W for the detection of pathology. CT is a digital X-ray investigation. Due to this, and somewhat paradoxically, white matter is depicted as being darker than gray matter because of the radiolucency of lipid-containing material.

Iodinated contrast material administered intravenously enhances blood within the cerebral arteries, veins, and dural venous sinuses. Enhancement is also seen in the highly vascular choroid plexuses and in those structures external to the blood–brain barrier such as the pituitary gland and infundibulum.

With MRI, the mechanism of enhancement with its own intravenous contrast agent, gadolinium DTPA, is quite different but, on T1W images, those structures which enhance become hyperintense (i.e., whiter) with similar appearances to CT. There are some important differences, however. Rapidly flowing blood is displayed as black "signal voids," a property shared with both air and cortical bone but for a different reason (paucity of protons) (Fig. 7.3). The role of angiography is primarily for the diagnosis and, in some cases, for the treatment of vascular abnormalities. Increasingly, non- or minimally invasive forms, magnetic resonance angiography (MRA) or CT angiography (CTA), are used for diagnosis. Depending on the technique, MRA may or may not require gadolinium DTPA. CTA necessitates an intravenous injection of iodinated contrast medium.

Catheter angiography, where iodinated contrast medium is injected directly into an artery (or vein), remains the gold standard. It is nearly always performed using digital subtraction, showing the vasculature in near isolation, free of bone detail.

The cervical carotid and vertebral arteries are usually cannulated via the femoral artery at the groin, although a brachial arterial approach can be used. The cervical carotid artery can be punctured directly but this time-honoured method is seldom used now. Angiographic interpretation is the province of the specialist neuroradiologist or clinical neuroscientist.

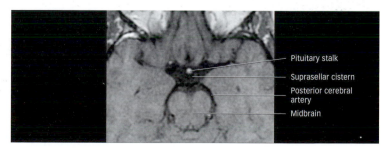

Fig. 7.3. **T1 weighted axial MRI after intravenous gadolinium DTPA. Suprasellar cistern.**

CT and MRI interpretation

The way in which a scan is "read" will be determined by the patient's suspected clinical diagnosis and the initial observations on the study. These same considerations will also influence the scan protocol and whether contrast agents are given. In any case, a sound appreciation of the normal appearances is essential.

First, the ventricular system should be assessed. Are the ventricles normal in size or enlarged? Is any enlargement part of generalised atrophy or is it obstructive? Are all the ventricles enlarged or, say, just the lateral ventricles, sparing the third and fourth? In this example, one would search for a lesion in the region of the foramen of Monro.

Next, one should look for abnormal density (CT) or signal intensity (MRI) within the cerebral substance, comparing the two sides. Is this associated with mass effect, manifest by sulcal effacement or distortion of the ventricles ("shift")? Examination of the basal CSF cisterns, with CT, will reveal subarachnoid hemorrhage, and their effacement is a vital clue to cerebral swelling. The appearance of the normal quadrigeminal plate cistern resembling a smile is reassuring (Fig. 7.2(g)).

Normal scan appearances alter with age. In the normal child, for instance, the cerebral ventricles and CSF cisterns can be very small. In the aging population, with some normal "volume loss," the CSF spaces may be prominent.

There are also "review areas" on scans, which repay a second look to identify a subtle change. For instance, on CT the interpeduncular cistern can harbor a small amount of subarachnoid blood. On MRI, the region of the posterior part of the third ventricle, cerebral aqueduct and pineal gland should be studied on the sagittal image. It is also the case that lesions seen easily on CT may not be clearly shown on MRI and vice versa. For example, a colloid cyst of the third ventricle can be difficult to see on MRI in its typical site at the foramen of Monro.

The skull (Fig. 7.4)

The skull vault or calvarium is formed from the frontal, temporal, parietal, and occipital bones. The skull vault consists of inner and outer bony "tables" or diploe separated by a diploic space containing marrow and large, thin-walled diploic veins. In children, marrow is typically "red," being active in blood production. It is hypointense on T1W MRI and, in the adult, is gradually replaced by "yellow" or fatty marrow, which becomes hyperintense on T1W images.

The bones of the vault are joined at various sutures, which consist of dense connective tissue. The sagittal suture joins the two parietal bones in the midline and the coronal suture joins them to the frontal bone.

In the infant there is a midline defect between the frontal and parietal bones at the junction of the sagittal and coronal sutures. This anterior fontanelle or bregma closes in the second year.

The occipital bone forms most of the walls and floor of the posterior cranial fossa, the largest of the three fossae. The single lambdoid suture separates the parietal and occipital bones. The clivus is formed from the basal portions of the sphenoid bone anteriorly and of the occipital bone posteriorly. The articulation is known as the basisphenoid synchondrosis and is also the site where the petrous apex joins the clivus.

Sutures are smooth in the newborn but throughout childhood, interdigitations develop followed by perisutural sclerosis (increased bone density) and ultimately fusion in the third or fourth decades or even later. However, for practical purposes sutural fusion occurs in adolescence because only in children does raised intracranial pressure, due for instance to a brain tumor, cause head enlargement.

Sutures must be distinguished from fractures of the skull and important features of the former include interdigitation, sclerosis and predictable positions.

The skull is invested in periosteum, both externally (pericranium) and internally (endosteum). The endosteum is firmly adherent to the connective tissues of the sutures.

The skull base is formed by contributions from the sphenoid, temporal, and occipital bones centrally and from the frontal and

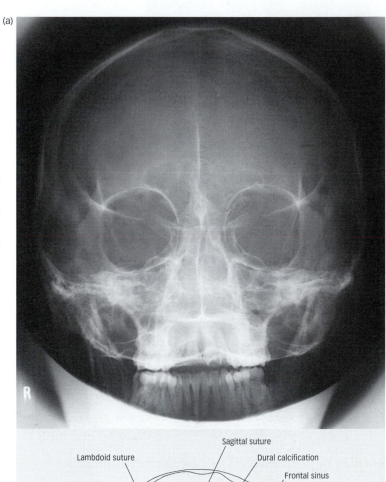

(a)

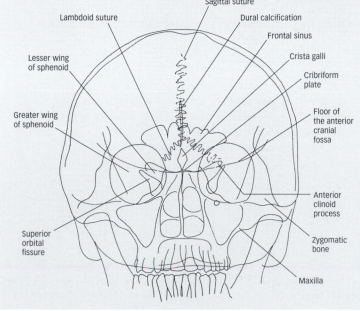

Fig. 7.4. **(a) Frontal, (b) lateral skull radiographs.**

accounts for the frequent occurrence of traumatic contusions in the inferior frontal lobes.

The sphenoid bone consists of a central body and greater and lesser wings. The greater wing forms the floor of the middle fossa. The lesser wing forms the posterior part of the anterior fossa and the "ridge," bordering the anterior part of the middle fossa. The body is pneumatized by the eponymous air sinus and bears the pituitary fossa on its superior surface.

A number of foramina occur in the skull base, transmitting a variety of structures and providing potential routes for the spread of extracranial disease (notably infection or tumor) into the vault (Fig. 7.5).

The foramina ovale, rotundum and spinosum are within the greater wing of the sphenoid bone. The foramina ovale and spinosum are often symmetrical, the foramen rotundum rarely so.

The foramen rotundum travels from Meckel's cave to the pterygopalatine fossa and transmits the maxillary (V2) division of the trigeminal nerve. On coronal CT it is identified inferior to the anterior clinoid processes. The foramen ovale transmits the mandibular (V3) division of the trigeminal nerve. On coronal CT it is identified inferior to the posterior clinoid processes (Figs. 7.6, 7.16).

The foramen spinosum is situated posterolateral to the larger foramen ovale and transmits the middle meningeal artery and vein.

The foramen lacerum contains cartilage and separates the apex of the petrous bone, the body of the sphenoid, and the occipital bone. It is crossed by the internal carotid artery.

The squamous portion of the temporal bone forms part of the lateral wall of the middle cranial fossa and its petromastoid constitutes part of the floor of the middle and posterior fossae. The occipital

Fig. 7.4. *Continued*

ethmoidal bones anteriorly. The inner surface of the skull base is divided into the anterior, middle, and posterior fossae. The anterior fossa is occupied by the frontal lobe; the middle fossa by the temporal lobe. The posterior fossa contains the brainstem and cerebellum.

The orbital plates of the frontal bones form most of the floor of the anterior fossa floor with a contribution from the ethmoid bone in the midline. The inner suface of the frontal bone, forming the floor of the anterior cranial fossa, has a relatively "rough" surface, which

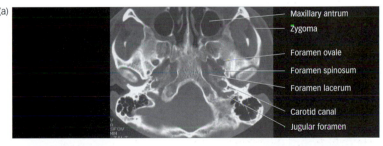
(a)

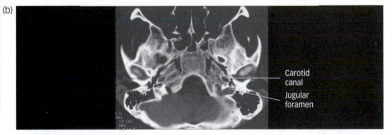
(b)

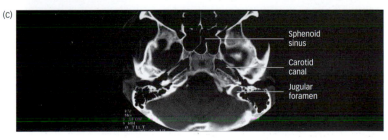
(c)

Fig. 7.5. **CT of the skull base: (a) to (c) are contiguous axial images, (a) the most inferior.**

(a)

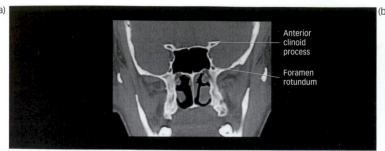

(b)

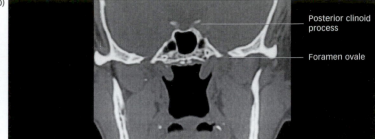

Posterior clinoid process

Foramen ovale

Anterior clinoid process

Foramen rotundum

Fig. 7.6. **Coronal CT of the skull base: (a) is anterior to (b).**

bone forms most of the floor and walls of the posterior fossa, the largest of the three.

The skull radiograph
Skull radiograph interpretation

Interpretation of skull radiographs (skull "series") can be challenging. It is relatively simple to obtain but is an insensitive indicator of intracranial pathology with roles limited to trauma and as a preliminary to cranial surgery. Of course, CT can largely meet these diagnostic requirements and, if necessary, a digital radiograph can be obtained as part of the CT examination.

Broadly, when confronted with a frontal radiograph, in the attempt to interpret the many overlapping and irregular lines and lucencies, it is helpful to compare the two sides. The lateral view gives a relatively clear view of the vault and pituitary fossa. One will also be influenced by the external clinical findings as to where an abnormality might be discovered. For practical purposes, the usual reason for requesting skull radiographs is to identify a fracture. There are normal vault "lucencies," which need to be considered, mainly due to blood vessel impressions, especially veins. A fracture will usually have a more distinct margin and, unlike blood vessels, does not often branch.

Normal calcifications may be encountered on skull radiographs arising in the pineal gland, choroid plexus, dura, and habenular commissure (Figs. 7.4, 7.17).

The brainstem (Fig. 7.7)

The brainstem consists of medulla, pons, and midbrain. The medulla, pons, and cerebellum together constitute the hindbrain.

The medulla commences at the foramen magnum as a continuation of the spinal cord. Initially it is "closed," possessing a central canal like the spinal cord. More superiorly, it becomes "open" as the central canal leads into the fourth ventricle. In the brainstem, the motor tracts are generally anterior to the sensory, hence the clinical usage of "anterior" columns meaning motor and "posterior" column, sensory. A number of decussations occur within the brainstem where both motor and sensory fibers cross the midline in accordance with the general principle that functional control of one-half of the body is largely exercised by the contralateral cerebral hemisphere. The sensory decussation is craniad to the motor, but both occur in the closed portion of the medulla.

The medulla leads superiorly into the pons, which has an anterior "belly" and a posterior tegmentum.

The midbrain has two cerebral peduncles transmitting the motor tracts. Its posterior portion is pierced by the cerebral aqueduct (of Sylvius), to connect the third and fourth cerebral ventricles.

(a)

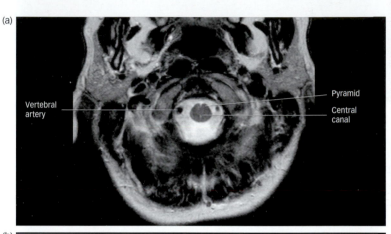

Pyramid

Central canal

Vertebral artery

(b)

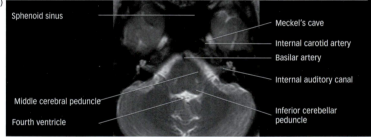

Sphenoid sinus

Meckel's cave

Internal carotid artery

Basilar artery

Internal auditory canal

Middle cerebral peduncle

Inferior cerebellar peduncle

Fourth ventricle

(c)

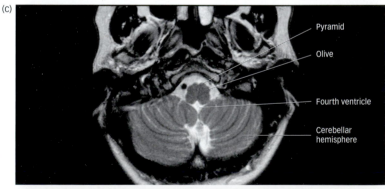

Pyramid

Olive

Fourth ventricle

Cerebellar hemisphere

(d)

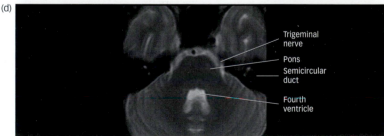

Trigeminal nerve

Pons

Semicircular duct

Fourth ventricle

Fig. 7.7. **T2 weighted axial MRI: (a) to (f), inferior to superior. The brainstem.**

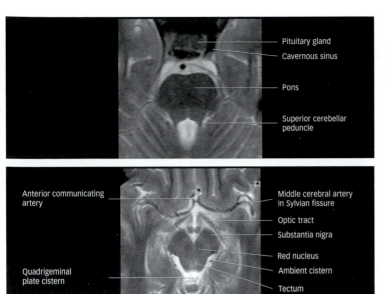

Pituitary gland
Cavernous sinus
Pons
Superior cerebellar peduncle

Anterior communicating artery
Middle cerebral artery in Sylvian fissure
Optic tract
Substantia nigra
Red nucleus
Ambient cistern
Quadrigeminal plate cistern
Tectum

Fig. 7.7. *Continued*

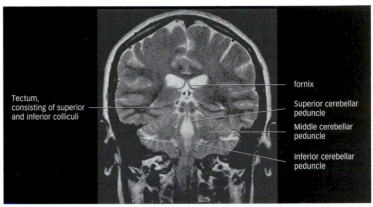

Tectum, consisting of superior and inferior colliculi
fornix
Superior cerebellar peduncle
Middle cerebellar peduncle
Inferior cerebellar peduncle

Fig. 7.8. **T2 weighted coronal MRI. The cerebellar peduncles.**

The posterior portion is known as the tectum or tectal plate. It consists of four colliculi or quadrigeminal bodies concerned with auditory and visual reflexes.

The cerebellum

The cerebellum consists of two hemispheres joined by a central vermis. The cortical mantle of the cerebellum overlies the white matter core as in the cerebral hemispheres but the cerebellar cortical ridges, known as the folia, and the intervening sulci are approximately parallel to one another and are linked to the brainstem by the paired cerebellar peduncles (Fig. 7.8). They are named logically. The inferior cerebellar peduncles join the medulla to cerebellum; the middle cerebellar peduncles (the largest), pons to cerebellum; the superior cerebellar peduncles, midbrain to cerebellum.

The cranial nerves

There are 12 paired cranial nerves, most of which are analogous to segmental nerves arising from the spinal cord. They variously provide sensory and motor nerves to structures in the extracranial head and neck and their distribution is complex.

The olfactory (first) cranial nerve consists of about 20 bundles of sensory nerves, which pass through the cribriform plate from the nose to the olfactory bulb inferior to the frontal lobe. The fibers pass posteriorly from the bulb along the olfactory tract and thence to the olfactory cortex.

The optic (second) cranial nerve is not a true nerve but rather an evagination (outpouching) of the brain. The nerve carries with it a meningeal sheath and is surrounded by CSF (Fig. 7.9). It passes, along with the ophthalmic artery, into the orbit through the optic canal.

The two optic nerves converge to form the optic chiasm, which lies in the suprasellar CSF cistern above the pituitary gland. From the chiasm, two optic tracts diverge toward the lateral geniculate bodies on each side of the midbrain. From there, the optic pathway continues through the temporal lobes towards the visual cortex in the occipital lobes.

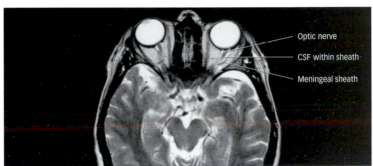

Optic nerve
CSF within sheath
Meningeal sheath

Fig. 7.9. **T2 weighted axial MRI. The optic nerve.**

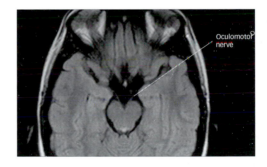

Fig. 7.10. **FLAIR axial MRI. The oculomotor nerve.**

Oculomotor nerve

The oculomotor (third) cranial nerve supplies the extraocular muscles with the exceptions of the lateral rectus and superior oblique. It arises in the midbrain from a nucleus at the level of the superior colliculi and emerges medial to the cerebral peduncle and is often seen on FLAIR sequence MR images (Fig. 7.10). It passes anteriorly between the posterior cerebral and superior cerebellar arteries to enter the superior part of the cavernous sinus and thence to the orbit through the superior orbital fissure, accompanied by the trochlear (fourth) and abducent (sixth) cranial nerves.

The oculomotor nerve is accompanied by parasympathetic fibers, which constrict the pupil. An intracranial aneurysm arising at the origins of either the posterior communicating or superior cerebellar arteries may result in an oculomotor palsy. This will be accompanied by dilatation of the pupil because the parasympathetic constrictor fibers travel peripherally in the nerve making them vulnerable to extrinsic pressure. The nerve also supplies levator palpebrae superioris – so that a third nerve palsy is associated with ptosis.

The trochlear (fourth) cranial nerve is the only one arising from the posterior surface of the brainstem, looping around the midbrain and passing with the oculomotor nerve between the superior cerebellar and posterior cerebral arteries. It is not seen on routine MRI scans.

The trigeminal (fifth) cranial nerve is the largest and most complex. The nerve arises from the pons and passes anteriorly to the trigeminal ganglion located in Meckel's cave at the posterior end of the cavernous sinus (Fig. 7.11).

The motor root, supplying the muscles of mastication, travels beneath the ganglion and exits the skull through the foramen ovale. The ophthalmic (V^I) division exits through the superior orbital fissure and the maxillary (V^{II}) division through the inferior fissure. The mandibular (V^{III}) division does not enter the cavernous sinus but exits inferiorly through the foramen ovale. The motor fibers to the muscles of mastication are confined to the mandibular divisions of the nerve.

The abducent (sixth) cranial nerve supplies the lateral rectus muscle and has a long intracranial course from pons to cavernous sinus, which makes it vulnerable in trauma to the skull base. The nerve may be seen on thin section MR images (Fig. 7.12).

The facial (seventh) cranial nerve, which innervates the muscles of facial expression, passes with the vestibulocochlear (eighth) cranial nerve from the pons to the internal auditory canal across the cerebellopontine angle cistern and these are routinely visualized on MRI (Fig. 7.12).

There is a sensory root, the intermediate nerve, which transmits secretomotor fibers to the lacrimal, submandibular, and sublingual glands and fibers conveying taste from the anterior two-thirds of the tongu (the chorda tympani).

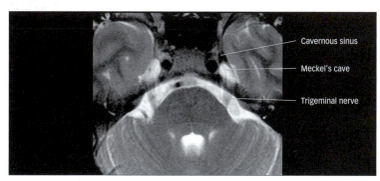

Fig. 7.11. **T2 weighted axial MRI. The trigeminal nerve.**

Cavernous sinus
Meckel's cave
Trigeminal nerve

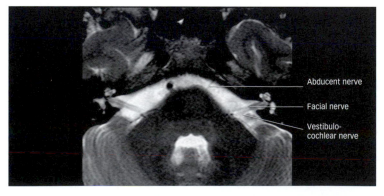

Fig. 7.12. **T2 weighted axial MRI. The abducent, facial and vestibulocochlear nerves.**

Abducent nerve
Facial nerve
Vestibulo-cochlear nerve

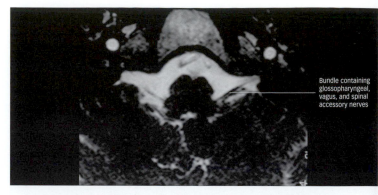

Fig. 7.13. **T2 weighted axial MRI. The glossopharyngeal, vagus and spinal accessory nerves.**

Bundle containing glossopharyngeal, vagus, and spinal accessory nerves

(a)

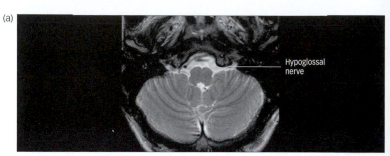

Hypoglossal nerve

(b)

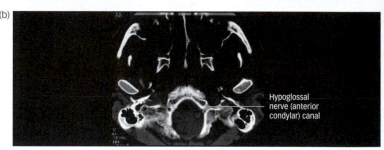

Hypoglossal nerve (anterior condylar) canal

Fig. 7.14. **(a) T2 weighted axial MRI, (b) Axial CT on bone algorithm. The hypoglossal nerve and canal.**

The glossopharyngeal (ninth), vagus (tenth) and spinal accessory (eleventh) cranial nerves are not seen on routine cranial MRI but can be resolved on special sequences. They arise from the medulla and form a bundle which leaves the cranium through the jugular foramen (Fig. 7.13).

The hypoglossal (twelfth) cranial nerve can be identified exiting through the hypoglossal, or anterior condylar, canal after emerging from the medulla between the olive and pyramid (Fig. 7.14). Again the nerve is not often seen on routine MRI.

The diencephalon, between the brainstem and cerebral hemispheres includes the thalamus, hypothalamus, and pineal gland, which all border the third ventricle. The thalami are paired, olive-shaped nuclear masses extending anteriorly as far as the foramen of Monro and forming most of the lateral walls of the third ventricle (Fig. 7.15). Medially, the thalami are apposed (not joined) at the massa intermedia or interthalamic adhesion. Laterally, the posterior limb of the internal capsule separates thalamus and lentiform nucleus. The posterior part of the thalamus is the pulvinar, which overlies the midbrain.

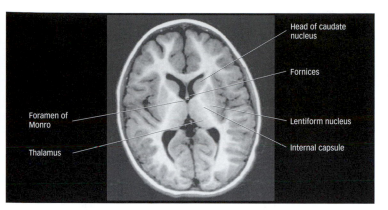

Fig. 7.15. **T1 weighted axial MRI. The basal ganglia.**

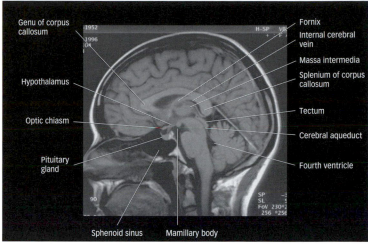

Fig. 7.17. **T1 weighted sagittal MRI. Showing the major midline structures.**

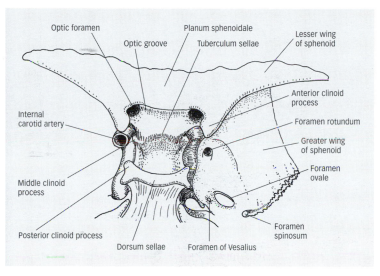

Fig. 7.16. **The bony anatomy of the sellar region.**

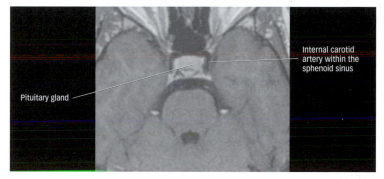

Fig. 7.18. **T1 weighted axial MRI after intravenous gadolinium DTPA. The cavernous sinuses.**

The hypothalamus forms the floor and part of the walls of the third ventricle. Posterior to the optic chiasm the pituitary stalk or infundibulum desscends to the pituitary gland. The tuber cinereum extends posteriorly from the stalk to the mamillary bodies, thence to the midbrain

The pituitary gland and perisellar region

The pituitary gland and perisellar region are frequently imaged in cases of endocrine disturbance, or in visual failure.

The pituitary gland lies in the sella turcica ("Turk's saddle") on top of the body of the sphenoid bone (Fig. 7.16). The body of the sphenoid bone contains the sphenoid air sinus, which provides a route for surgical access to the pituitary gland via the nose. The sella is roofed by the dural diaphragma sellae, which is pierced by the pituitary stalk leading to the hypothalamus (Fig. 7.17).

There is no blood–brain barrier around the pituitary gland, which therefore takes up intravenous contrast media avidly, either the iodinated agents used for CT or gadolinium DTPA used in MRI.

The pituitary gland should be no more than 9 mm in height, although it varies in size. In some normal individuals it appears as a thin rim of tissue at the base of the sella. Its upper margin is usually concave, although it is often convex in children and in females of reproductive age.

The cavernous sinuses lie lateral to the sella on either side (Fig. 7.18). These are extradural venous spaces through which the internal carotid arteries pass, and damage to the artery here, due to trauma, can result in a carotico-cavernous fistula.

The third, fourth, branches of the fifth and the sixth cranial nerves pass through the cavernous sinus to the orbit. The cavernous sinuses receive blood from a number of facial veins and venous plexuses providing a potential route for sepsis to spread intracranially (Fig. 7.27).

Above the pituitary gland is the appropriately named suprasellar or chiasmatic CSF cistern, which contains the circle of Willis and the optic chiasm (Fig. 7.19). The basal ganglia are part of the extrapyramidal system and consist of the caudate and lentiform nuclei, together known as the corpus striatum, the amygdala, and claustrum.

The caudate nucleus is C-shaped with a head indenting the frontal horn of the lateral ventricle, a body running alongside the body of the lateral ventricle and a tail lying just above the temporal horn of the lateral ventricle.

The lentiform nucleus is divided in the parasagittal plane into the medial globus pallidus and larger lateral putamen.

The motor and sensory tracts

The upper motor neurones controlling voluntary movement are found in the precentral gyrus of the frontal lobe. Axons pass from the cell

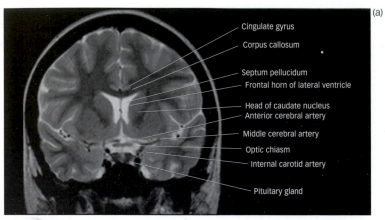

Fig. 7.19. **T2 weighted coronal MRI. The pituitary gland and suprasellar cistern.**

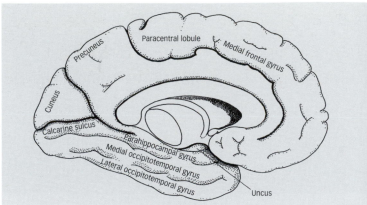

(a)

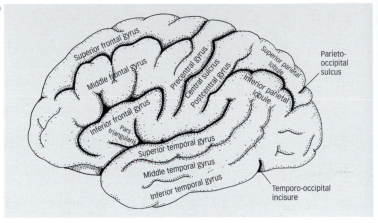

(b)

Fig. 7.20. **The cortical gyri: (a) medial and (b) lateral aspects.**

bodies via the corona radiata to the internal capsule to the motor nuclei in the brainstem and to the anterior horns of the spinal cord.

The internal capsule is a V-shaped myelinated tract with the genu (bend) pointing medially separating the anterior and larger posterior limbs.

From the various cutaneous receptors, sensory neurones with cell bodies in the dorsal root ganglia synapse in the thalami. Axons of second-order neurones synapse in the thalami. Third-order neurons pass from thalami to sensory cortex.

The cerebral hemispheres

The cerebral hemispheres lie above the tentorium and are divided by fissures and sulci into frontal, parietal, temporal, and occipital lobes. The limbic system (see below) is also considered to be a lobe.

The hemispheres are linked by the corpus callosum, the largest of the commissural tracts, which interconnect paired structures across the midline. Other examples of commissural tracts are the anterior, posterior, and habenular commissures. The anterior and posterior commissures are landmarks used in image-guided neurosurgical procedures.

The corpus callosum is a myelinated tract and appears curved in sagittal images. The anterior rostrum blends with the anterior commissure inferiorly. The curved genu (knee) leads posteriorly to the body thence the largest and most posterior part, the splenium. Fibers from the corpus callosum sweep anteriorly into the frontal white matter as the forceps minor and posteriorly into the occipital white matter as the forceps major.

There is considerable individual variation in gyral anatomy but the more constant gyri are shown in Fig. 7.20. It is also important to appreciate that the relationship of function to structure may be variable and that speech, for example, may be represented over a number of gyri with intervening white matter. Equally, it may be difficult to identify the central sulcus and adjacent motor strip accurately. In specialized centers, functional MRI is carried out with patients performing appropriate intellectual, motor, or sensory tasks. Regional variations in cerebral oxygen utilization can then be registered and the eloquent area identified.

The anatomical boundaries of the individual lobes may be indistinct, depending on the aspect. The frontal lobe is the largest of the anatomical lobes occupying the anterior cranial fossa and extending posteriorly

to the central sulcus. In common with the temporal lobe, the frontal lobe has three major gyri, superior, middle, and inferior, which are oriented horizontally. The temporal lobe occupies the middle cranial fossa The anterior limit of the parietal lobe is the central sulcus, which, running in the coronal plane, separates the precentral (motor) gyrus of the frontal lobe from the postcentral (sensory) gyrus. The boundary between the parietal and temporal lobes laterally is indistinct but the parieto-occipital incisure medially defines the two lobes. The main cortical supply of the occipital lobe relates to vision. The calcarine (visual) cortex can be seen to indent the posterior (occipital) horns of the lateral ventricles. The cortex here is deeply infolded with little intervening white matter. Inferiorly and laterally the temporo-occipital fissure marks the division between the two lobes.

The Sylvian or lateral fissure separates the superior surface of the temporal lobe from the inferior frontal lobe and the anterior parietal lobe. During development, the cortex overlying the basal ganglia is invaginated to form the insula (Fig. 7.21). The cortex in front of, above, and below this depression expands to form covering folds termed the operculum.

The Sylvian fissure is formed between these folds. On axial imaging it runs in the coronal plane on the lower cuts and in the sagittal plane on the higher slices. On coronal MRI, it resembles the shape of a T lying on its side.

The limbic system

The anatomy of the limbic system is complex, its many components retaining their descriptive, classical names, unfortunately with some

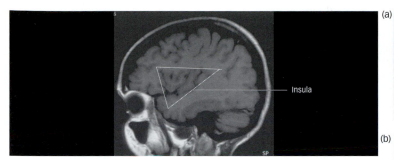

Fig. 7.21. **T1 weighted parasagittal MRI. The insula.**

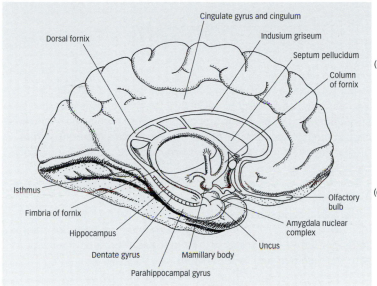

Fig. 7.22. **Medial aspect of cerebral hemisphere showing the limbic system.**

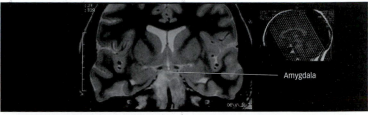

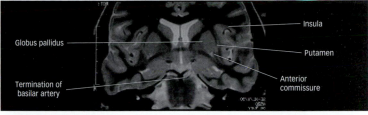

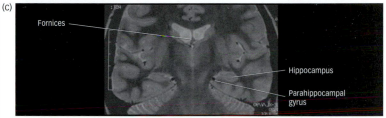

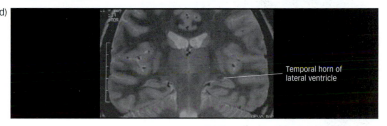

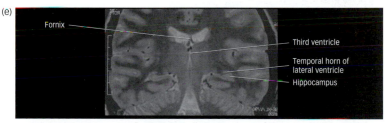

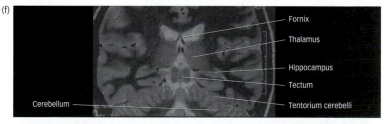

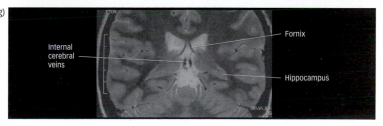

Fig. 7.23. **T2 weighted extended coronal MRI. Obtained perpendicular to the long axes of the temporal lobes, (a) to (h), anterior to posterior.**

synonyms. The limbic system is also classified as one of the cerebral lobes (the limbic lobe).

The limbic system can be regarded as two C-shaped gyral arches in each hemisphere, running from near to the midline in the frontal lobes to the medial part of the temporal lobe (Fig. 7.22). Their course mirrors the curved relationship of the frontal and temporal lobes and the various components can be identified in Fig. 7.23.

The arches comprise the following.

The outer limbic gyrus (the larger arc)

subcallosal area, cingulate gyrus, parahippocampal gyrus, subiculum, uncus,

The inner limbic gyrus (the smaller arc)

supracallosal and paraterminal gyri, hippocampus, The outer and inner limbic gyri are separated by the hippocampal sulcus and its continuation, the callosal sulcus.

The hippocampus (sea horse or monster), consists of a head, body, and tail, and is the first part of the cerebral cortex to form (Figs. 7.24, 7.25). The broadest part is the head anteriorly. More posteriorly, the body of the hippocampus forms the floor of the temporal horn of the lateral ventricle. The tail extends around the splenium of the corpus callosum and is continuous with the supracallosal indusium griseum. The indusium griseum is closely applied to the surface of the corpus callosum and anteriorly it merges with the paraterminal gyrus.

(h)

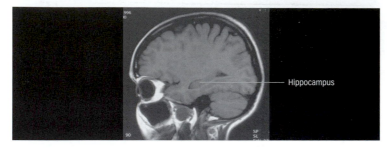

Quadrigeminal plate cistern

Splenium of corpus callosum

Fig. 7.23. *Continued*

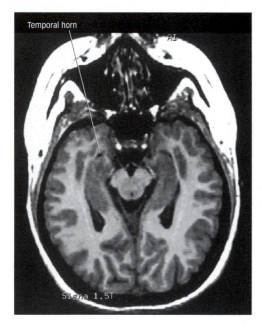

Hippocampus

7.24. **T1 weighted parasagittal MRI. The hippocampus.**

Temporal horn

Sigma 1.5T

Fig. 7.25. **T1 weighted axial image in the plane of the temporal lobe. The hippocampus.**

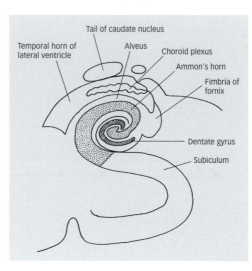

Fig. 7.26. **Diagram of components of limbic lobe.**

Tail of caudate nucleus
Temporal horn of lateral ventricle
Alveus
Choroid plexus
Ammon's horn
Fimbria of fornix
Dentate gyrus
Subiculum

The internal structure of the hippocampus is complex and beyond the resolution of MRI at the time of writing. The dentate gyrus and cornu Ammonis infold into one another in the form of interlocking Us (Fig. 7.26).

The parahippocampal gyrus is inferior to the hippocampus and forms the inferomedial aspect of the temporal lobe. Superior to it is the hippocampal fissure and laterally, the collateral sulcus. The parahippocampal gyrus becomes continuous with the cingulate gyrus which continues anteriorly into the subcallosal area.

The subiculum is a cortical layer of the parahippocampal gyrus and is separated by the hippocampal fissure from the dentate gyrus.

The most anterior part, the hippocampal head, is separated by the temporal horn of the lateral ventricle from the amydala (almond), which lies more anteriorly and a little superiorly.

Axons from the subiculum and hippocampus form the alveus (white matter) and converge as the fimbria, which leads into the fornix (arch) at the posterior hippocampus. The two fornices converge near to the foramen of Monro. The uncus is formed anteriorly from the parahippocampal gyrus and posteriorly from the medial part of the hippocampal head.

The subcortical structures of the limbic system comprise the amygdala, habenula, mamillary body, and septal nuclei.

The septal area is in the medial part of the frontal lobes and includes the subcallosal area and paraterminal gyri, from the outer and inner limbic gyri, respectively. There are also limbic connections with the thalamus and hypothalamus.

The cerebral envelope (Fig. 7.27)

The meninges invest the brain and spinal cord. The three constituent parts are the outer, fibrous dura mater, the avascular, lattice-like, arachnoid mater, and the inner vascular layer, the pia mater.

The subarachnoid space contains the cerebrospinal fluid (CSF), which surrounds the cerebral arteries and veins. It is situated between the arachnoid, which bridges the sulci, and the pia, which is closely applied to the cerebral surface.

The dura consists of two layers which separate to enclose the venous sinuses (Fig. 7.27). The outer layer is the periosteum of the inner table of the skull. The inner layer covers the brain and gives rise to the falx and tentorium.

The falx cerebri is a sickle-shaped fold of dura, which forms an incomplete partition between the cerebral hemispheres. The superior and inferior sagittal sinuses mark its upper and lower margins.

The "point of the sickle" is anterior, the falx being broader posteriorly. When there is swelling of one hemisphere, subfalcine herniation "midline shift" will be more pronounced anteriorly as a result.

The tentorium cerebelli ("tent") forms a roof over the contents of the posterior fossa. Anteriorly and superiorly, the tentorial hiatus constitutes a gap in the tent through which the midbrain passes. The free medial edge of the tentorium extends anteriorly to form the lateral wall of the cavernous sinus on each side.

On axial CT, the anterior margin of the tentorium migrates medially on the higher scans. Structures lateral to the line are supratentorial, structures medial to the line are infratentorial (or lie within the posterior fossa).

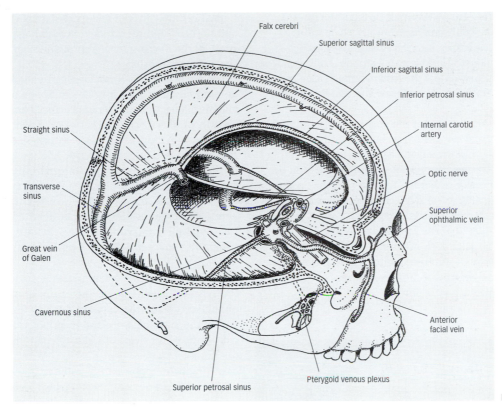

Falx cerebri
Superior sagittal sinus
Inferior sagittal sinus
Inferior petrosal sinus
Internal carotid artery
Optic nerve
Superior ophthalmic vein
Anterior facial vein
Pterygoid venous plexus
Superior petrosal sinus
Cavernous sinus
Great vein of Galen
Transverse sinus
Straight sinus

Fig. 7.27. **The cranial dura.**

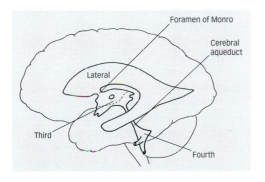

Foramen of Monro
Cerebral aqueduct
Lateral
Third
Fourth

Fig. 7.28. **The cerebral ventricles.**

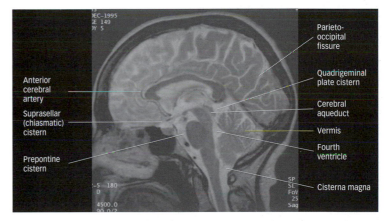

Anterior cerebral artery
Suprasellar (chiasmatic) cistern
Prepontine cistern
Parieto-occipital fissure
Quadrigeminal plate cistern
Cerebral aqueduct
Vermis
Fourth ventricle
Cisterna magna

Fig. 7.29. **T2 weighted sagittal MRI. The basal CSF cisterns.**

The cerebral ventricular system cerebrospinal fluid spaces (Fig. 7.28)

The cerebral ventricular system consists of the paired lateral and single third and fourth ventricles.

Cerebrospinal fluid (CSF), is produced in the choroid plexuses, and most of it is in the lateral ventricles, entering medially through the choroidal fissures. It flows from the lateral ventricles to the third ventricle through the foramen of Monro, in the anterior portion of the roof of the third and from the third to fourth via the cerebral aqueduct of the midbrain. From the fourth ventricle, the CSF enters the subarachnoid spaces, leaving through the paired foramina of Luschka, laterally and the midline, single foramen of Magendie. These foramina provide a potential route of spread for intraventricular tumors.

At the base of the brain, there are relatively large CSF spaces, the basal CSF cisterns, which are important both anatomically and in CT or MRI diagnosis. Although named individually, according to adjacent structures, they interconnect freely with each other and with the CSF spaces generally (Figs. 7.29, 7.3, 7.7(f)).

The cerebral blood circulation

Cerebral arteries

The brain is supplied with oxygenated blood by the paired internal carotid and vertebral arteries. The common carotid artery in the neck divides at the approximate level of the upper border of the thyroid cartilage (C4) into its internal and external branches, the latter supplying the various craniofacial structures.

The internal carotid artery

The internal carotid artery is the larger of the two branches, receiving 70% of the common carotid blood flow. It lies posterolateral to the external carotid near to the bifurcation and neither common nor internal carotid arteries have cervical branches.

The internal carotid artery enters the skull through the carotid canal and courses anteromedially and horizontally (the petrous segment) before turning superiorly into the cavernous sinus (Fig. 7.5). In this position the artery forms the shape of a siphon. Emerging from the cavernous sinus, the artery enters the subarachnoid space and divides into its terminal branches, the anterior and middle cerebral arteries (Fig. 7.19).

There are no angiographic markers of the position of the intracavernous portion of the internal carotid artery, but the origin of the ophthalmic artery is usually within the subarachnoid space (Fig. 7.30).

The posterior communicating artery passes on each side from the internal carotid to the posterior cerebral arteries.

The anterior choroidal artery arises from the internal carotid artery just above the posterior communicating artery

The circle of Willis is situated in the suprasellar cistern and links the internal carotid arteries with each other and with the vertebrobasilar system, via the single anterior and paired posterior communicating arteries. It affords some protection in the event of occlusion of major arteries by facilitating "cross-flow."

Most cerebral arterial aneurysms are borne on the circle of Willis and so their rupture results in hemorrhage into the subarachnoid space in the first instance. This includes an aneurysm at the origin of the ophthalmic artery

The circle of Willis is not circular in shape but rather a five- or six-pointed star, (Fig. 7.31). It is also complete in only a minority of individuals. Indeed, the intracranial arterial anatomy is subject to so many (usually minor) variations that a broad picture will be given here.

The terminal branches of the internal carotid artery are the anterior and middle cerebral arteries. The anterior cerebral artery passes horizontally towards the midline and links to the other anterior cerebral by the anterior communicating artery, (Figs. 7.1(h), 7.2(e)). This first part is known as the A1 segment. From the origin of the anterior communicating artery both anterior cerebral arteries next turn superiorly and run in close proximity, above the corpus callosum, following a curving path posteriorly, again near the midline (Fig. 7.29).

The middle cerebral artery passes horizontally and laterally towards the Sylvian fissure. There is then a division into two or three branches (middle cerebral artery bifurcation or trifurcation). These ascend within the Sylvian fissure and then loop infreolaterally over the opercular cortex over the cerebral surface to supply the parietal and temporal lobes.

Arising from the proximal anterior and middle cerebral arteries, a leash of small, perforating arteries (the lenticulostriates) supplies a variety of structures including the basal ganglia and internal capsule.

The vertebral arteries are the first branches of the subclavian arteries. They ascend vertically within the foramina transversaria of the 6th to the 2nd cervical vertebrae and posterolaterally through the foramen transversarium of the atlas, (first cervical vertebra). The arteries then travel superomedially to pass into the skull through the foramen magnum, piercing the dura and entering the subarachnoid space (Figs. 7.7 (a, b)). At the level of the pontomedullary junction, the two arteries join to form the midline basilar artery (Figs. 7.1 (a)–(f), 7.2 (c)–(e)), which runs anterior to the brainstem. The cerebellum is supplied by the posterior inferior cerebellar arteries, arising from the vertebral arteries just before the confluence, and the anterior inferior- and superior cerebellar arteries, arising from the basilar artery.

(a)
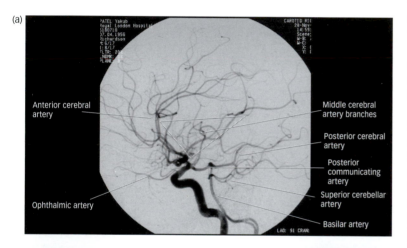

(b)
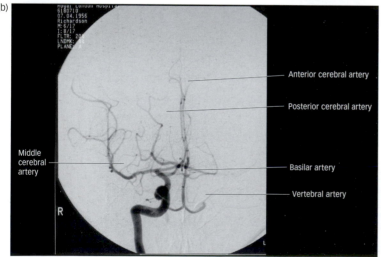

Fig. 7.30. **Internal carotid angiograms: (a) lateral, (b) frontal projections. Although only the internal carotid artery has been injected with contrast medium, the vertebrobasilar system and contralateral middle cerebral artery are opacified due to the Circle of Willis. The triangle in (a) encloses the proximal middle cerebral artery branches. Note that the anterior ceebral arteries are near to the midline, whereas the middle cerebral artery branches are laterally situated.**

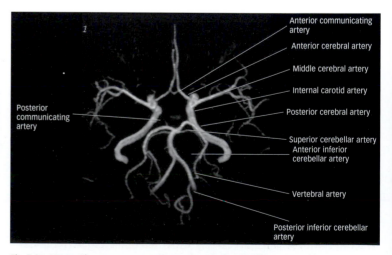

Fig. 7.31. **Magnetic resonance angiography. Circle of Willis.**

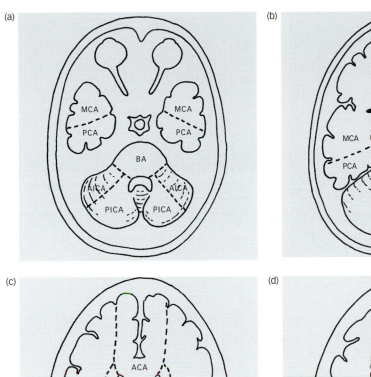

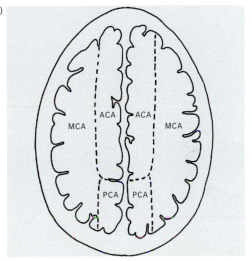

Fig. 7.32. **The vascular territories.**

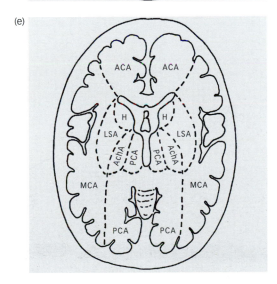

pass posteriorly to the brainstem. It is also the case that similar very small arteries arise from all of the major intracerebral arteries, including the communicators.

Vascular territories

Knowledge of the cerebral arterial territories can be of assistance in the identification of a lesion as an infarct. These are illustrated in Fig. 7.32.

Cerebral venous drainage

A complex venous system drains blood from the brain into the internal jugular veins in the neck (Fig. 7.33).

The superficial veins over the cerebral surface drain into the dural venous sinuses, venous spaces within the dura (Fig. 7.27). There is also a deep system draining into the paired internal cerebral veins (Figs. 7.2(i), 7.8, 7.17, 7.23(g)). The internal ceebral veins lead into the single great vein of Galen, thence into the straight sinus. This venous "confluence" is situated in the quadrigeminal plate cistern. Another confluence, this time, of the dural venous sinuses occurs at the internal occipital protuberance or torcula, where the superior sagittal, transverse and straight sinuses converge.

The terminal branches of the basilar artery are the posterior cerebral arteries, which supply the occipital (visual) cortex (Figs. 7.2 (g), 7.23 (b)). Many smaller branches arise from the basilar arteries, which are too small to be shown at angiography. These "perforating" arteries (a), (b)

(c)

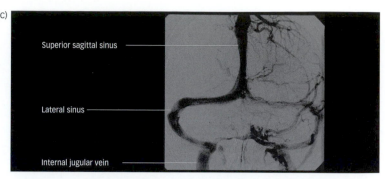

Superior sagittal sinus

Inferior sagittal sinus

(a)

(b)

Internal cerebral vein   Great vein of Galen   Straight sinus

Internal jugular vein

Transverse sinus

Sigmoid sinus

Superior sagittal sinus

Lateral sinus

Internal jugular vein

Fig. 7.33. **The cerebral venous system: (a) T1 weighted sagittal MRI after intravenous gadolinium DTPA; (b) carotid angiogram, venous phase, lateral view; (c) carotid angiogram, venous phase, frontal view. Note that the lateral sinuses are not seen on the MRI because it is a midline "slice." The angiograms represent a 3-D arrangement displayed in 2-D.**

CLAUDIA KIRSCH

Imaging considerations

The bony orbit is best examined with CT and images acquired in the coronal plane are particularly useful to identify fractures. The radiation dose to the lens is not insignificant and cataract formation is a potential hazard

Plain radiography of the orbit is largely reserved for identifying metallic intraocular bodies prior to MRI scanning.

Intraorbital fat is hypodense (dark) on CT scans and provides a useful contrast to the other soft tissue structures within the orbit. Conversely fat is hyperintense (white)on both T1- and T2-weighted MRI. The relative brightness of fat can obscure the orbital contents and, to counter this "fat-suppressed" MR, pulse sequences are used, usually in combination with intravenous gadolinium DTPA. These render fat hypointense (dark) and thus improve visualization of the globe, extraocular muscles, and lacrimal gland. Overall, the soft tissue detail with MRI is superior to CT.

Anatomy of the bony orbit

The orbital cavity is shaped like a pyramid with its apex posteromedially and base anterolaterally, opening onto the face. It is represented diagrammatically in Fig. 8.1. The bony margins separate it from the anterior cranial fossa and frontal air sinus superiorly, the ethmoid and sphenoid air sinuses medially, the maxillary sinus inferiorly, and the temporal fossa laterally (Fig. 8.2).

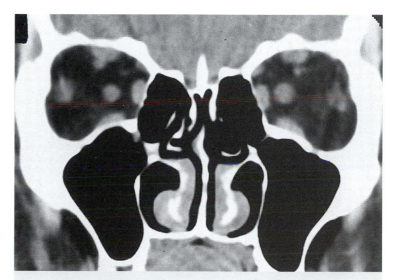

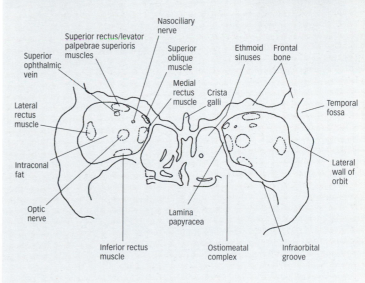

Fig. 8.2. **Coronal CT scan to show the orbital wall and extraocular muscles.**

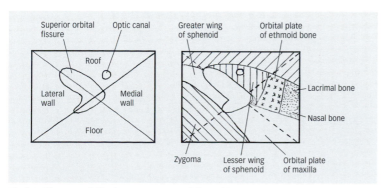

Fig. 8.1. **Diagram of the bony anatomy of the orbit.**

The triangular orbital floor, which slants laterally, and the rectangular medial orbital wall, the descriptively named lamina papyracea, are both thin. The floor also has a groove running anteriorly to a canal, the infraorbital foramen, transmitting the infraorbital nerve, contributing further to its potential weakness. Predictably both the medial wall and floor are prone to fractures and are demonstrated optimally by coronal CT scans.

The lateral wall, also triangular is the thickest and is formed largely from the zygomatic bone.

At the orbital apex, the optic canal, contained within the lesser wing of the sphenoid bone, transmits the optic nerve, sympathetic fibers and ophthalmic artery, opening posteriorly into the middle cranial fossa (Fig. 8.3).

The superior orbital fissure (SOF), is located inferior and lateral to the optic canal and is separated from the optic canal by the optic strut (Fig. 8.4). The SOF is formed superiorly by the lesser wing of the sphenoid bone and inferiorly by the greater wing. The SOF transmits the oculomotor (IIIrd), trochlear (IVth), and abducent (VIth) cranial nerves, the terminal ophthalmic nerve branches, and ophthalmic veins.

Seen from the front, the inferior orbital fissure (IOF), forms a V-shape with the SOF, its apex pointing medially.

The SOF communicates posteriorly with the cavernous sinus and the IOF with the pterygopalatine fossa, which leads to the infratemporal fossa. The veins crossing these fissures thus provide possible routes for the spread of orbital infections both intracranially and into the deep facial structures.

The periorbita is composed of the bony orbit periosteum and serves as a protective barrier against spread of infection or neoplasms. Posteriorly it merges with the optic nerve dura. Anteriorly, the periorbita continues as the orbital septum inserting on the tarsi within each of the eyelids. Each tarsus is a fibrous structure, one in the upper, one in the lower eyelid. In the upper eyelid, the orbital septum also joins the tendon of the levator palpebrae muscle.

A preseptal orbital infection in front of the orbital septum may be managed medically. A postseptal infection has spread behind the septal barrier with loss of the normal orbital tissue planes and is at risk for subperiosteal, intracavernous, and intracranial extension.

Soft tissues of the orbit

The soft tissues of the orbit are embedded in a fatty reticulum. The globe is approximately 2.5 cm in diameter (Fig. 8.5). It is situated

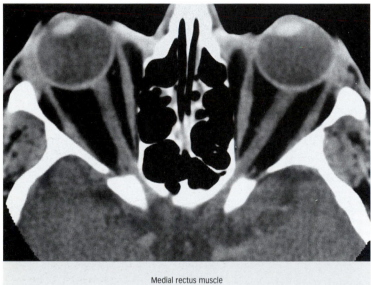

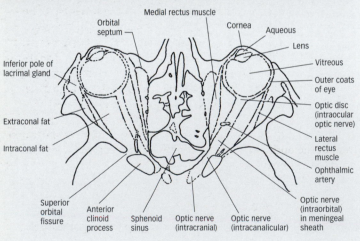

Fig. 8.3. **Axial CT scan at the level of the optic canals.**

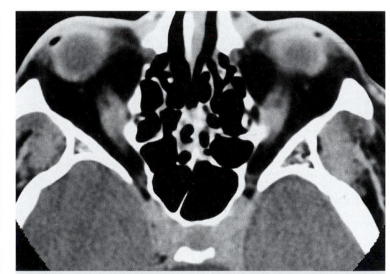

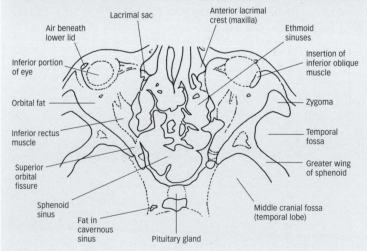

Fig. 8.4. **Axial CT scan (inferior to Fig. 8.3), at the level of the superior orbital fissure.**

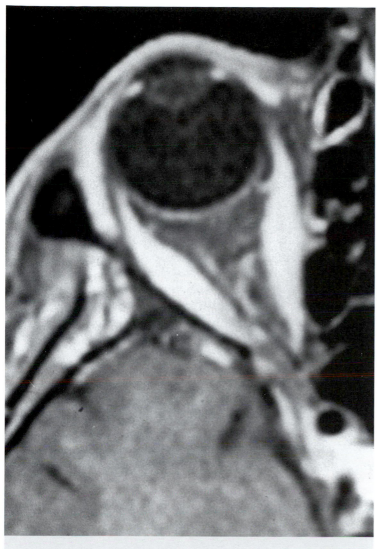

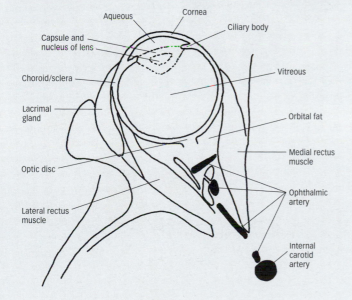

anteriorly within the orbit and has three coats enclosing its contents. From the outside in, there are the tough, fibrous sclera, the vascular, pigmented choroid, and the retina. These cannot be resolved separately on routine CT and MRI. The vascular choroid can be identified as a "blush" during carotid angiography.

Anteriorly within the globe, the circumferential ciliary body supports the lens and, anterior to the lens, the iris.

The lens demarcates two compartments, the anterior aqueous and posterior vitreous. The iris further divides the aqueous (incompletely because of the pupil), into anterior and posterior chambers. The cornea forms the anterior boundary of the anterior chamber.

The episcleral membrane, or Tenon's capsule, encapsulates the posterior four-fifths of the globe, dividing it from the posterior orbital fat.

The optic nerve

The optic nerve is not a true cranial nerve. Rather, it is a cerebral white matter tract. It arises from the posterior globe and pursues an undulating course within the rectus muscle cone to pass through the optic canal accompanied by the ophthalmic artery (Fig. 8.6). Each optic nerve is about 4.5 mm in diameter and 5 cm long. The distance from the posterior globe to the optic canal is about 2 cm. This redundancy permits the nerve mobility with the eye movements.

Belying its nature the optic nerve is surrounded by cerebrospinal fluid and encased in a meningeal sheath.

The extraocular muscles

Six striated extraocular muscles, four rectus muscles, and two oblique muscles are responsible for the eye movements. The extraocular muscles are arranged as a cone and define intra- and extraconal compartments.

The four rectus muscles arise from the annulus of Zinn, a tendinous ring at the optic foramen. The annulus is composed of four extraocular muscles: superior rectus, medial rectus, and inferior, and lateral rectus muscles (Fig. 8.2). The oblique muscles have a more complex course. The superior oblique muscle, the longest and thinnest of all orbital muscles, originates from the sphenoid bone periosteum extending along the superior medial orbital wall as a slender tendon. The muscle enters the trochlea (L. pulley), a small fibrocartlaginous ring, sharply turning posterolaterally and inferiorly behind the superior rectus muscle inserting on the lateral sclera. The inferior oblique muscle originates from the medial portion of the anterior orbital floor and is inserted into the lateral aspect of the eyeball.

The triangular levator palpebrae superioris muscle arises above and in front of the optic canal to pass forwards above superior rectus to insert into the upper eyelid.

The nerves of the orbit

The superior oblique muscle is supplied exclusively by the trochlear (IVth) cranial nerve and lateral rectus by the abducent (VIth) cranial

Fig. 8.5. **Fat-suppressed T1W axial MRI to show the globe.**

nerve. The oculomotor (IIIrd) cranial nerve supplies the remaining, striated, extraocular muscles. Sensory innervation is via the ophthalmic division and maxillary divisions of the trigeminal (Vth) cranial nerve.

The lacrimal gland

The almond-shaped lacrimal gland is located anterolaterally in the roof of the orbit in a small fossa (Fig. 8.7). It forms tears, which diffuse to the conjunctiva and drain via the tear ducts running in the medial portions of the margins of the upper and lower lids.

The orbital vasculature

The main arterial supply of the orbit is via the ophthalmic artery, which arises directly from the internal carotid artery, in the majority of cases just after it has exited the cavernous sinus (Fig. 8.8). It passes forward to enter the orbit through the optic canal, accompanying the optic nerve within the dural sheath. Initially inferior to the nerve, the ophthalmic artery crosses the nerve to lie medial to it (Fig. 8.9). It gives off numerous branches within the orbit including the central artery of the retina. Further arterial supply is provided by branches of the external carotid artery.

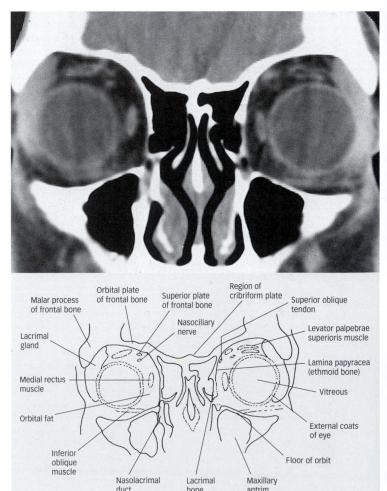

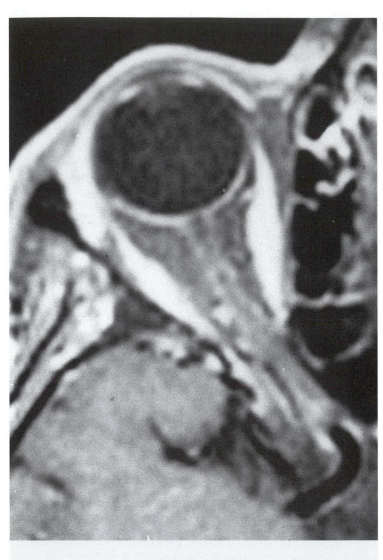

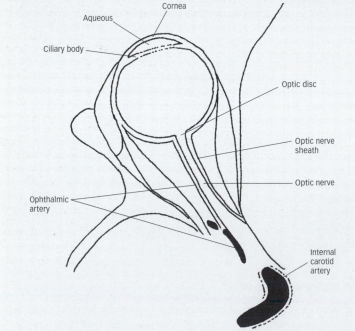

Fig. 8.6. **Fat-suppressed T1W axial MRI to show the optic nerve.**

Fig. 8.7. **Coronal CT scan (anterior to Fig. 8.2), to show the lacrimal glands.**

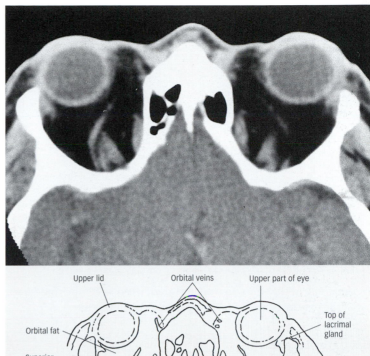

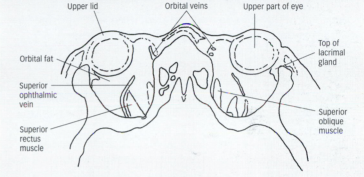

Fig. 8.10. **Axial CT scan (superior to Fig. 8.9), to show the superior ophthalmic veins.**

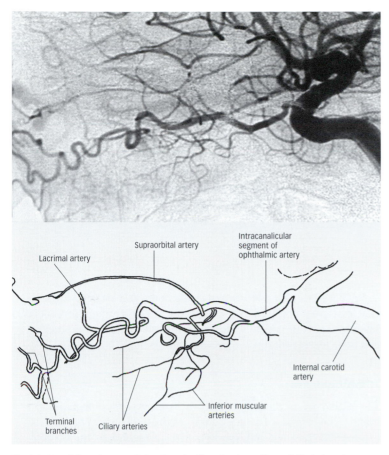

Fig. 8.8. **Carotid angiogram, lateral projection, to show the ophthalmic artery.**

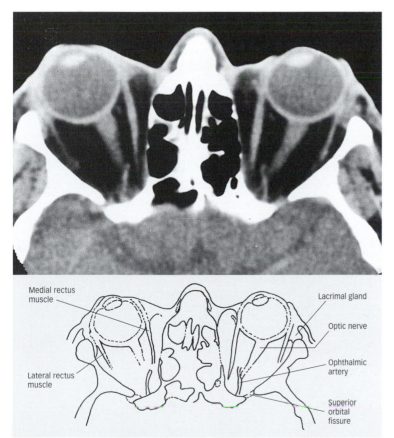

Fig. 8.9. **Axial CT scan to show the ophthalmic arteries.**

There are two major veins within the orbit. Both are valveless. The superior ophthalmic vein forms posteromedial to the upper eyelid, from facial veins. It courses posteriorly, close to the ophthalmic artery, to enter the cavernous sinus through the superior orbital fissure (Fig. 8.10).

The inferior ophthalmic vein forms in the anterior orbital floor and usually joins the superior ophthalmic vein.

The optic pathways

The optic nerves extend posteriorly from the optic canal, ascending medially at a 45 degree angle. They then then fuse to form the optic chiasm, which is superior to the pituitary gland and may be compressed by a large pituitary tumor extending upwards. From the optic chiasm the two optic tracts pass posterolaterally (refer to Fig. 8.1(g),(h), see Chapter 7 Figs. 7.17, 7.90). These then merge with the hemispheres, becoming indistinguishable on routine CT or MRI. Visual fibers pass posteriorly through the temporal lobes to the visual cortex within the occipital lobes, thus running a long intracranial course.

CLAUDIA KIRSCH

The anatomy of the ear is conveniently described as comprising three parts: the external ear, the middle ear, and the inner ear.

The external ear

The external ear consists of the pinna or auricle and the S-shaped external auditory canal, extending from the auricle to the tympanic membrane.

The outer third of the external auditory canal is fibrocartilagenous and contains numerous hairs and glands for producing cerumen. The inner two-thirds are bony and contains few hairs or cerumen glands.

The tympanic membrane separates the external auditory canal from the middle ear and is embedded in the bone of the tympanic ring. It is

in two parts: a smaller, looser and thicker pars flaccida superiorly, and a larger, tenser, fibrous pars tensa inferiorly. The scutum represents the superior tympanic ring to which the tympanic membrane is attached. It is particularly well seen on coronal thin section CT (Fig. 9.1).

The middle ear

The middle ear, or tympanic cavity, is a treasure trove of spaces, bumps, and recesses. The lateral wall of the tympanic cavity is formed almost completely by the tympanic membrane and is subdivided into three spaces relative to it: from above down, the epitympanum (syn. the attic or epitympanic recess), mesotympanum, and hypotympanum.

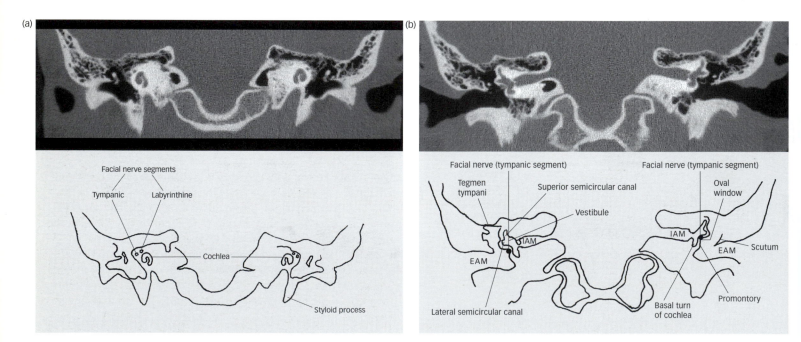

Fig. 9.1. **Coronal HRCT, the petrous bone, (a) is anterior to (b).**

Applied Radiological Anatomy for Medical Students. Paul Butler, Adam Mitchell, and Harold Ellis (eds.) Published by Cambridge University Press. © P. Butler, A. Mitchell, and H. Ellis 2007.

The epitympanum is located above the tympanic membrane. The mesotympanum is at the same level as the tympanic membrane and the hypotympanum is located below it.

The roof of the middle ear cavity is known as the tegmen tympani, which separates the tympanic cavity below from the middle cranial fossa above. The floor also consists of a thin plate of bone below which is the bulb (superior part) of the internal jugular vein.

A bony wall separates the tympanic cavity medially from the inner ear. In the epitympanum is a prominence due to the lateral semicircular canal and, inferior to this prominence, is the facial nerve canal. On the medial wall also, but more anterior and just opposite the tympanic membrane, is the cochlear promontory, created by the large first turn of the cochlea. The medial wall also contains two small windows. Above the promontory, the oval window is apposed by the footplate of the stapes, vibrations from which are transmitted to the inner ear. Located inferior to the oval window and below the

promontory is the round window, closed by a secondary tympanic membrane, allowing for counter pulsation of the perilymph fluid.

From the anterior wall of the tympanic cavity, the pharyngolympanic (Eustachian) tube travels anteromedially to open into the pharynx (Fig. 9.2). On the posterior wall is a prominent ridge, the pyramidal eminence, in which there is an aperture transmitting the stapedius tendon. Lateral to the pyramidal eminence is the facial nerve recess, medial to it the sinus tympani.

The posterior wall of the tympanic cavity has a superior opening, the aditus ad antrum (Fig. 9.3). This leads posteriorly from the epitympanic recess into the mastoid air cells and is a pathway for the spread of disease between the middle ear and mastoid process.

Within the middle ear cavity is the ossicular chain consisting of the descriptively named malleus (L. hammer), incus (L. anvil), and stapes (L. stirrup), each connected by synovial joints (Figs. 9.4 and 9.5).

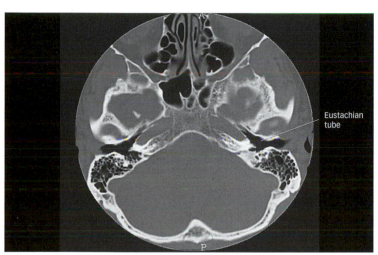

Fig. 9.2. **Axial HRCT to show the eustachian or pharyngotympanic tubes.**

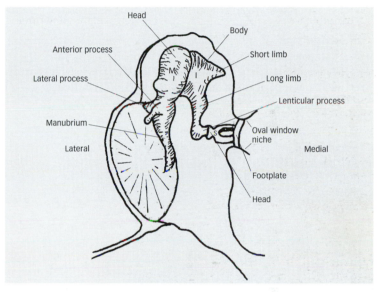

Fig. 9.4. **Diagram of the auditory ossicles.**

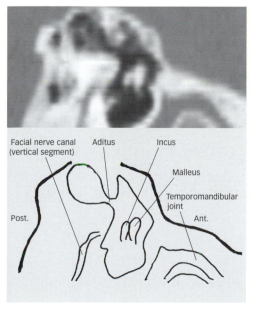

Fig. 9.3. **HRCT reformatted in the sagittal plane to show the aditus ad antrum.**

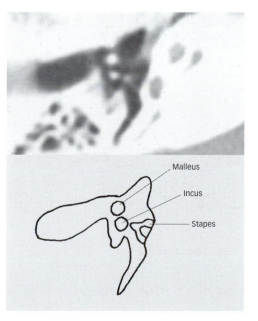

Fig. 9.5. **Axial HRCT showing the ossicular chain.**

The malleus has a lateral short process and manubrium embedded within the tympanic membrane, and head and neck, best seen on thin section coronal CT images. A small diathrodial joint exists between the malleus and incus within the attic.

The largest ossicle is the incus, posterior to the malleus (Fig. 9.3), composed of a body, with a short process extending posteriorly acting as a fulcrum allowing the incus to rotate. The incus has a lenticular and a long process meeting at about a 90-degree angle.

The cup-shaped lenticular process connects to the ball-shaped head of the stapes (capitulum) via a tiny cartilaginous disc, forming a tiny synovial diathrodial communication. The stapes footplate is attached to the oval window via an annular ligament.

The best way to see the ossicular chain is on thin section axial and coronal CT bone windows.

Two important muscles protect the ossicles from loud noises.

The stapedius muscle, supplied by facial (VIIth cranial) nerve, stretches the annular ligament of the stapes. It arises from the pyramidal eminence and attaches to the stapes footplate.

The tensor tympani muscle, supplied by the trigeminal (Vth cranial) nerve, dampens sounds by tightening the tympanic membrane. The tensor tympani muscle lies parallel and medial to the eustachian tube. It sits in a bony sulcus, extending from the pyramidal eminence anteriorly to attach on to the stapes footplate.

The inner ear

The inner ear or vestibulocochlear organ is responsible for hearing and balance. It is well protected and contained within the petrous portion of the temporal bone. The bony labyrinth of the inner ear encloses the membranous labyrinth, which contains fluid known as endolymph.

The bony labyrinth comprises the cochlea, vestibule, and semicircular canals and is best appreciated on CT (Figs. 9.1 and 9.6). The cochlea (L. snail shell), is anterior to the vestibule and semicircular canals. It is shaped like a spiral seashell, making two and half turns around its bony central core called the modiolus (L. nave of the wheel), which has small openings for blood vessels and nerves. The bony labyrinth encloses the membranous labyrinth, which comprises the saccule and utricle (not visible on imaging), contained within the vestibule, three semicircular ducts, located within the three semicircular canals, and the cochlear duct located within the cochlea. These sacs and ducts contain endolymph and are end organs for hearing (cochlea) and balance (semicircular canals). Between the bony labyrinth and the membranous labyrinth is fluid known as perilymph. Because these are fluid-containing structures, they are best visualized on MRI, using T2-weighted sequences (Figs. 9.7 and 9.8).

The vestibule communicates posteriorly with the semicircular canals and with the posterior fossa via the vestibular aqueduct. The vestibular aqueduct contains the endolymphatic duct, which extends through posterior cranial fossa into a blind pouch, called the

Fig. 9.7. **Coronal T2 weighted MRI through the cochleae.**

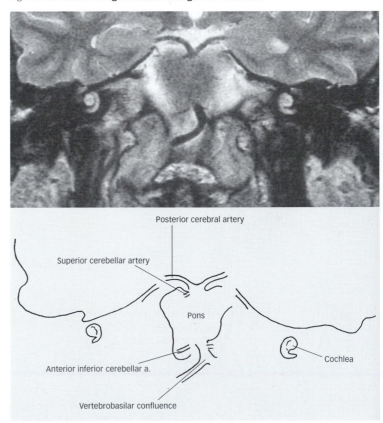

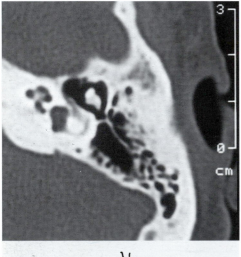

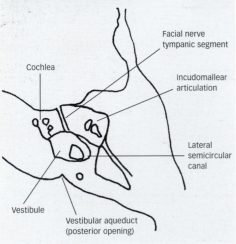

Fig. 9.6. **Axial HRCT showing the bony labyrinth.**

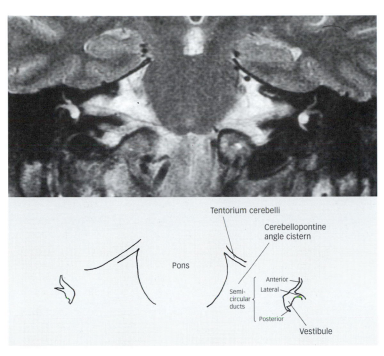

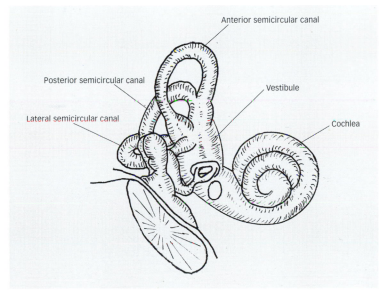

Fig. 9.8. **Coronal T2 weighted MRI through the vestibules.**

Fig. 9.9. **Diagram of the bony labyrinth.**

endolymphatic sac, located below the dura mater along the posterior petrous temporal bone.

The three semicircular canals (Fig. 9.9) are superior and posterior to the vestibule, with which they communicate. They are arranged at right angles to one another as the superior (anterior), horizontal (lateral), and posterior semicircular canals. There are only five entrances into the vestibule because the superior and posterior canals share a common limb (the common crus). The anterior or superior semicircular canal is at a right angle to the long axis of the petrous temporal bone. The posterior semicircular canal runs parallel to the axis of the petrous temporal bone in close relation to the sigmoid

sinus. The horizontal semicircular canal is located just above the facial nerve canal in the middle ear.

The internal auditory canal

The internal auditory canal or meatus (IAM) is separated laterally from the inner ear via a thin plate of bone, containing openings for the facial (VIIth cranial) nerve and the vestibulocochlear (VIIIth cranial) nerve. The internal auditory canal is a round opening into the posterior cranial fossa and is divided into quadrants. The bony crista falciformis divides the IAM horizontally. Bill's bar divides the canal vertically. The facial (VIIth cranial) nerve is located anteriorly and superiorly. The cochlear division of the eighth nerve is located anteriorly and inferiorly. Located in the posterior canal are the superior and inferior quadrants and the remaining divisions of the eighth nerve, the superior and inferior vestibular nerves.

The facial nerve

The facial nerve follows a complex course within the petrous bone. It may therefore be damaged by trauma to the petrous bone, including surgery, and by, for example, middle ear infections.

It arises from the brainstem and crosses the cerebellopontine angle cistern in an anterolateral direction, accompanying the vestibulocochlear (VIIIth cranial) nerve into the internal auditory meatus (Fig. 9.10). The facial nerve then enters its canal turning more anteriorly towards the geniculate ganglion (the labyrinthine portion), (Fig. 9.11). It then turns sharply posterolaterally, at the fist genu (L. knee) to course along the medial wall of the middle ear cavity (the tympanic portion) just below the lateral semicircular canal and above the oval window niche (Fig. 9.1). At the second genu, the facial nerve makes a second sharp turn, descending vertically to exit via the stylomastoid foramen in the mastoid bone (Fig. 9.3) dividing in the parotid gland into five branches supplying the muscles of facial expression.

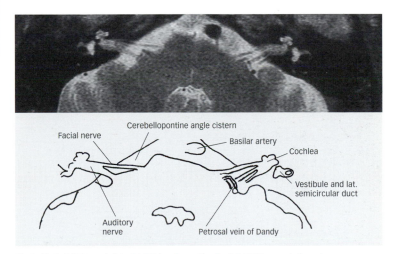

Fig. 9.10. **Axial T2 weighted MRI to show the facial (VIIth cranial) and vestibulocochlear (VIIIth cranial) nerves within the internal auditory meatus.**

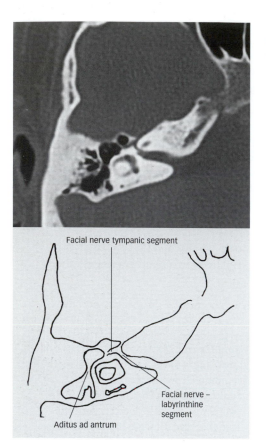

Fig. 9.11. **Axial HRCT to show the facial nerve canal**.

Facial nerve tympanic segment

Facial nerve – labyrinthine segment

Aditus ad antrum

The cerebellopontine angle cistern

The cerebellopontine angle cistern is one of the large, interconnecting cerebrospinal fluid spaces (cisterns) at the base of the brain. It is a subarachnoid space whose medial margin is the pons, and whose lateral margins include the posterior petrous bone. Traversing the cistern are the facial (VIIth cranial) and the vestibulocochlear (VIIIth cranial) nerves. The anterior–inferior cerebellar artery, (AICA), a loop from which can occasionally enter the IAM, the petrosal vein of Dandy and the trigeminal (Vth cranial) nerve may also occur within the cistern.

Section 4 | The head, neck, and vertebral column

Chapter 10 | The extracranial head and neck

JUREERAT THAMMAROJ
and JOTI BHATTACHARYA

The facial skeleton and musculature

For imaging, the skull and facial bones are best considered as a whole (Fig. 10.1). For descriptive purposes, they are usually divided into the upper face, consisting of the supraorbital ridge and frontal bone; the midface extending from the supraorbital margin to the upper jaw; and the lower face comprising the mandible.

Plain radiographs are still commonly performed. The occipito-mental or Water's view (Fig. 10.2), occipito-frontal (Fig. 10.3) and lateral views (Fig. 10.4) are the usual projections. Increasingly, 3-D CT is supplanting radiographs for facial trauma. CT is also ideal for examining the skull base, pterygopalatine and infratemporal fossae (Fig. 10.5).

The mandible and temporomandibular joint

The mandible (Fig. 10.6) is the strongest of the facial bones and is particularly well shown by dental panoramic radiography (or orthopantomography) (Fig. 10.7). The teeth are borne by the inferior alveolar process. The mandibular foramen lies on the inner surface of the ramus and admits the inferior alveolar nerve (trigeminal) into the mandibular canal, which opens on the outer surface of the mandible as the mental foramen.

The muscles of the tongue and floor of the mouth are attached to the inner surface of the body of the mandible. The powerful muscles of mastication insert on the ramus and angle.

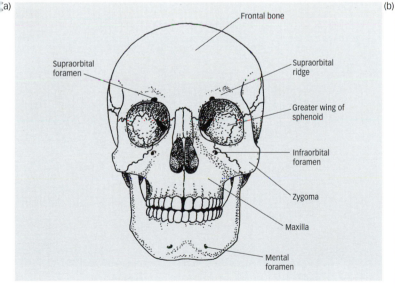

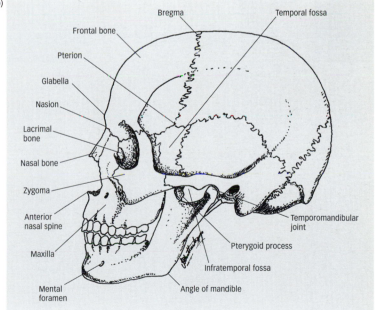

Fig. 10.1(a),(b). **Diagram of skull and facial skeleton. (a) frontal view, (b) lateral view.**

Applied Radiological Anatomy for Medical Students. Paul Butler, Adam Mitchell, and Harold Ellis (eds.) Published by Cambridge University Press. © P. Butler, A. Mitchell, and H. Ellis 2007.

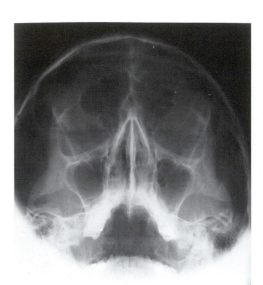

Fig. 10.2. **Occipito-mental radiograph (Water's view). The petrous ridges should be projected just below the maxillary antra. This is the best single view for the antra. Note the lucency of the canal for the posterior superior alveolar nerve in the lateral antral wall.**

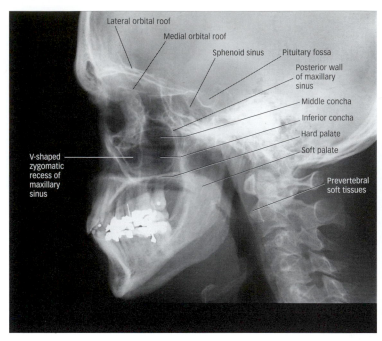

Fig. 10.4. **Lateral radiograph of facial bones. Note the V-shaped shadows of the zygomatic recesses of the maxillary antra and the shadows of the middle and inferior turbinates. The posterior walls of both antra are visible.**

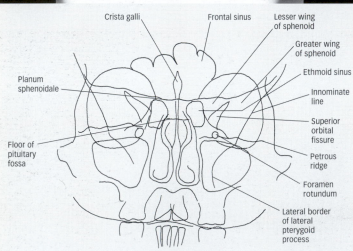

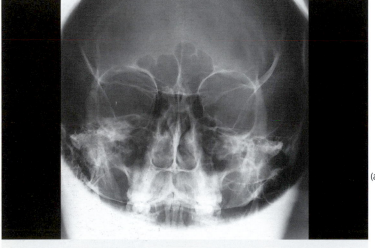

Fig. 10.3. **Occipito-frontal radiograph (Caldwell view). The petrous ridges should be projected over the lower third of the orbit. This is the best frontal view for the ethmoid and frontal sinuses. Note the foramen rotundum always lying immediately below the superior orbital fissure.**

(a)

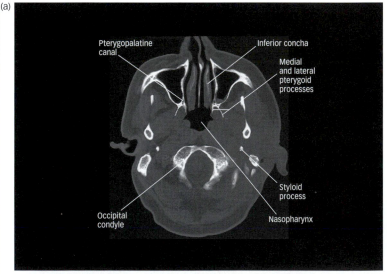

Fig. 10.5(a)–(g). **Series of CT images of skull base demonstrating the pterygopalatine and infratemporal fossae and related anatomy. Images are contiguous from inferior to superior. The lowest scan (a) shows the pterygopalatine canal which communicates with the mouth. The sphenopalatine foramen is seen in (e) opening into the nasal cavity posterior to the middle turbinate. The horizontal canals of the foramen rotundum (g) and the vidian (pterygoid) canal (e) link the fossa to the middle cranial fossa and the foramen lacerum, respectively. The lateral opening of the pterygopalatine fossa into the infratemporal fossa is called the pterygomaxillary fissure.**

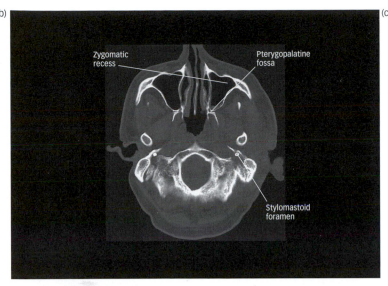

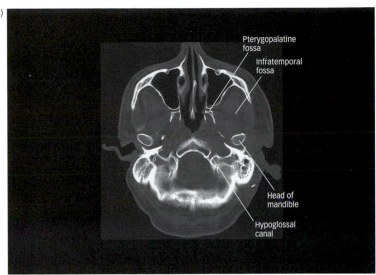

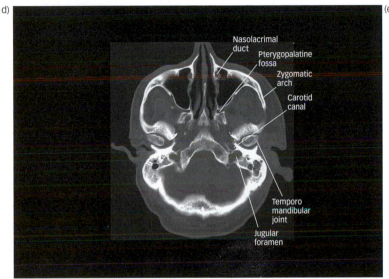

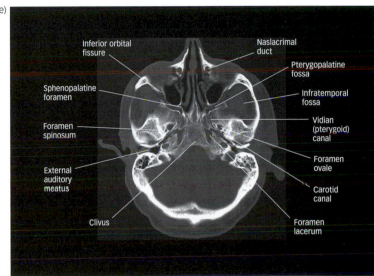

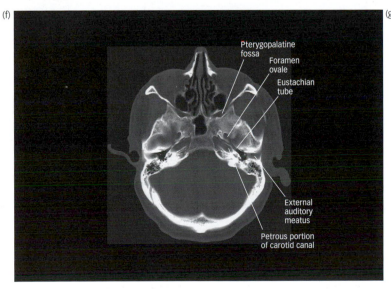

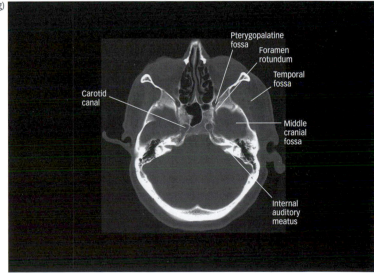

Fig. 10.5(a)–(g). *Continued*

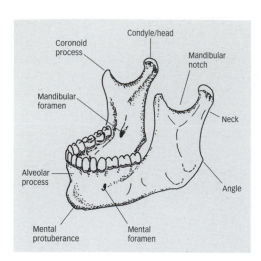

Fig. 10.6. **Diagram of mandible. The masseter and medial pterygoid muscles insert on the outer and inner aspects of the angle. The lateral pterygoid muscle inserts on the neck and the temporalis inserts on the coronoid process.**

communicate via the choanae with the nasopharynx posteriorly, and laterally with the paranasal sinuses. This region is best demonstrated by CT (Fig. 10.5). The nasal cavity is roofed in its mid-portion by the cribriform plate of the ethmoid bone which is perforated by about 20 foramina for the olfactory nerve, and ethmoidal vessels. The hard palate forms the floor. The lateral wall is complex bearing the three turbinates (or conchae) and their corresponding meatuses (Fig. 10.8).

The paranasal sinuses and ostiomeatal complex

The paranasal sinuses (frontal, maxillary, ethmoid, and sphenoid) arise as outgrowths of the nasal cavity and communicate with the cavity via ostia. Although well seen on radiographs (Figs. 10.2–10.4), their anatomy and pathology is best appreciated on coronal CT images.

The pyramid-shaped maxillary sinus, or antrum, lies within the body of the maxilla (Fig. 10.9). The roots of the molar and premolar teeth may project into the sinus but are usually covered by a thin layer of mucosa. Posteriorly lies the pterygopalatine fossa. The maxillary ostium is in the superior part of the medial wall and opens into the ethmoid infundibulum, a narrow channel between the uncinate process and the ethmoid bulla. This in turn opens into a curved groove in the middle meatus below the ethmoid bulla: the hiatus semilunaris (Fig. 10.8(b)). The frontal sinus opens into the anterior end of this groove, with the ethmoid cells opening more posteriorly. These structures, known as the ostiomeatal complex, form the drainage pathway for secretions from the sinuses; obstruction here

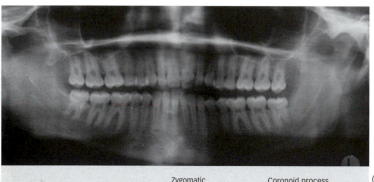

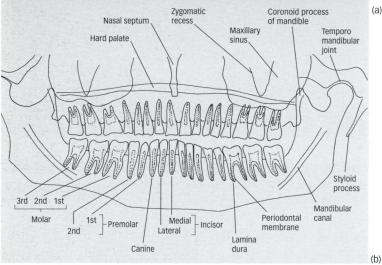

(a)

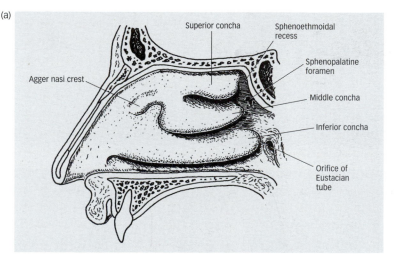

Fig. 10.7. **Orthopantomography, or dental panoramic radiograph of the mandible and maxilla. This technique in which the X-ray tube and film cassette rotate synchronously and reciprocally around the patient's head gives a good survey of the upper and lower jaws.**

The mandibular condyle articulates with the mandibular fossa of the temporal bone at the temporomandibular joint (TMJ) (Fig. 10.5 (c)–(e)).

Nasal cavity

The external nose consists of superior bony and inferior cartilaginous portions. The nasal cavity extends from the skull base to the roof of the mouth and is divided by the nasal septum into two fossae, which

(b)

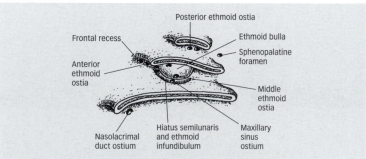

Fig. 10.8(a),(b). **Diagrams of lateral wall of nasal fossa, (a) before and (b) after removal of the turbinates to expose the underlying meati. Note that only the posterior ethmoid cells open into the superior meatus and only the nasolacrimal duct opens into the inferior meatus.**

(a)

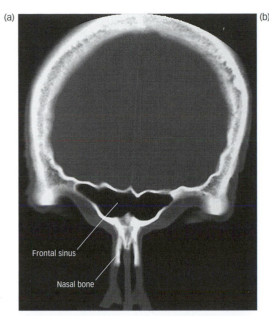

Frontal sinus

Nasal bone

(b)

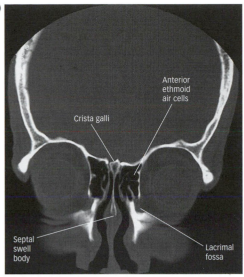

Anterior ethmoid air cells

Crista galli

Septal swell body

Lacrimal fossa

Fig. 10.9(a)–(f). Coronal CT series on bone window settings demonstrating the anatomy of the paranasal sinuses and ostiomeatal complex from anterior (a) to posterior (f).

(c)

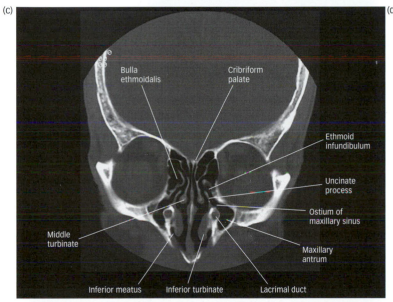

Bulla ethmoidalis

Cribriform palate

Ethmoid infundibulum

Uncinate process

Ostium of maxillary sinus

Maxillary antrum

Middle turbinate

Inferior meatus

Inferior turbinate

Lacrimal duct

(d)

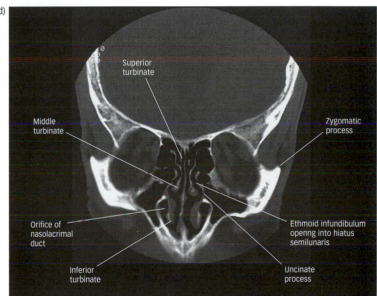

Superior turbinate

Middle turbinate

Zygomatic process

Ethmoid infundibulum openng into hiatus semilunaris

Orifice of nasolacrimal duct

Inferior turbinate

Uncinate process

(e)

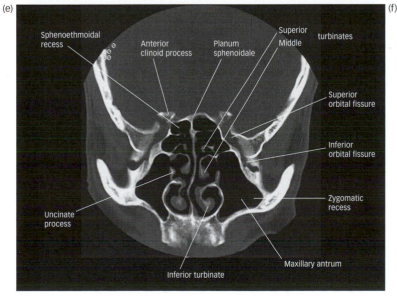

Sphenoethmoidal recess

Anterior clinoid process

Planum sphenoidale

Superior Middle turbinates

Superior orbital fissure

Inferior orbital fissure

Zygomatic recess

Uncinate process

Inferior turbinate

Maxillary antrum

(f)

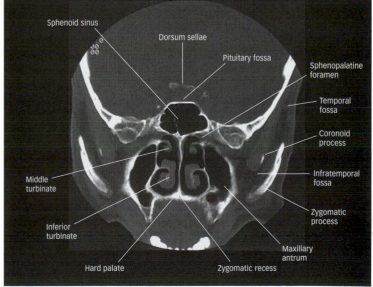

Sphenoid sinus

Dorsum sellae

Pituitary fossa

Sphenopalatine foramen

Temporal fossa

Coronoid process

Infratemporal fossa

Zygomatic process

Maxillary antrum

Middle turbinate

Inferior turbinate

Hard palate

Zygomatic recess

thus has a pivotal role in the development of sinusitis and endoscopic sinus surgery seeks to clear these obstructions.

The oral cavity tongue and salivary glands

The oral cavity contains the teeth, tongue and salivary glands, while posteriorly lies the pharynx. The mylohyoid muscles (originating from the mandible and inserting on the hyoid bone) form the "diaphragma-oris," which divides the floor of the mouth into a sublingual space superomedially and a submandibular space inferolaterally (Fig. 10.10). The tongue is a muscular organ, supplied by the hypoglossal nerve and readily identified on CT and MRI.

The parotid gland is the largest of the three, and lies over the ramus of the mandible and masseter muscle (Fig. 10.11) with its deep portion curling around the mandible. It is traversed by the facial nerve which divides here into its five terminal branches. The course of the nerve divides the gland into superficial and deep lobes. The facial nerve is seldom visible on imaging studies, although its course can be traced. The fatty structure of the parotid gives it a CT density between that of muscle and fat. On MRI scans, the gland is hyperintense to muscle.

The submandibular gland is the principal structure in the submandibular space. Because the gland wraps around the posterior border of the mylohyoid, its deep portion lies in the sublingual space. Its CT density is approximately that of muscle and higher than that of the parotid gland. It shows strong contrast enhancement.

The sublingual gland is the smallest of the major salivary glands lying anterior to the submandibular gland.

(a)
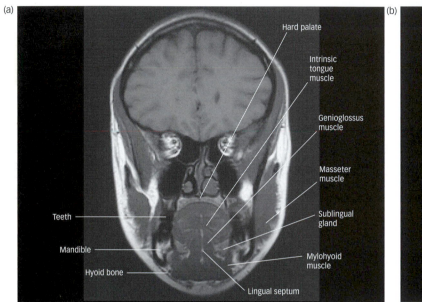
(b)

Fig. 10.10. **T1W MRI of the head coronal (a) and sagittal (b) demonstrating the structures of the floor of the mouth and tongue.**

(a)
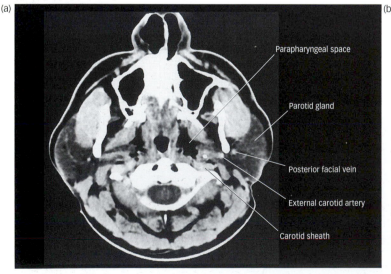
(b)
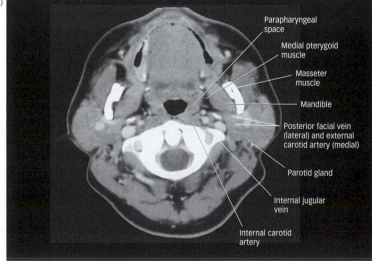

Fig. 10.11(a),(b). **Contrast-enhanced axial CT through the parotid gland. Note the typical attenuation of the adult parotid gland in (a), intermediate between fat and muscle density. In children and some adults the parotid can almost be isodense with muscle (b) which can make identification of mass lesions difficult.**

The pharynx

The pharynx is a fibromuscular tube, which forms the upper part of the aerodigestive tract and extends from the skull base to the lower border of the cricoid cartilage where it becomes continuous with the oesophagus. It is divided into the nasopharynx, oropharynx, and laryngopharynx (Fig. 10.12) and consists of mucosal, submucosal, and muscular layers. Posteriorly lies the prevertebral fascia. The major function of the pharynx is swallowing, which can be studied by videofluoroscopy.

Pharyngeal morphology and adjacent structures are well shown by cross-sectional techniques. The nasopharynx is closely related to the foramina of the central skull base, accounting for the frequency of neurological involvement in invasive nasopharyngeal carcinomas (Fig. 10.13).

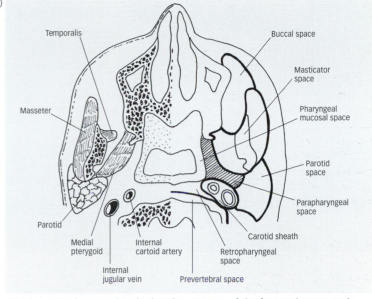

(a)

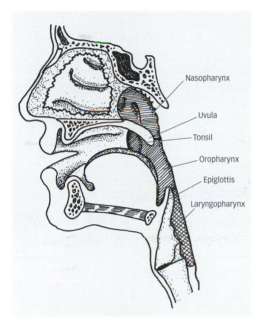

Fig. 10.12. **Diagram of subdivisions of pharynx.**

Fig. 10.14. **Parapharyngeal and other deep spaces of the face and upper neck:** (a) schematic diagram through the nasopharynx showing the deep spaces of the face on the right and some of their contents on the left. The central position of the parapharyngeal space (shaded) is emphasised. (b)–(d) contiguous axial T1W MRI superior to inferior demonstrating the high-signal fatty triangle of the parapharyngeal space.

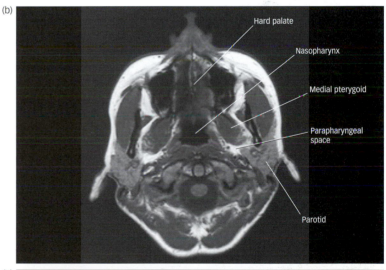

(b)

Fig. 10.13. **Coronal CT through nasopharynx showing the pharyngeal recesses.** Also demonstrated are the foramen rotundum superolaterally, and the vidian canal linking the pterygopalatine fossa and the foramen lacerum, inferomedially.

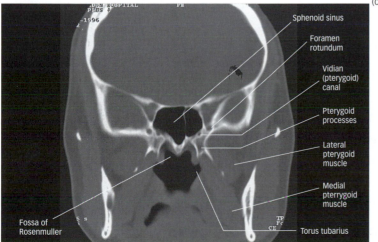

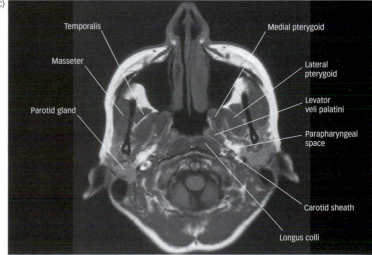

(c)

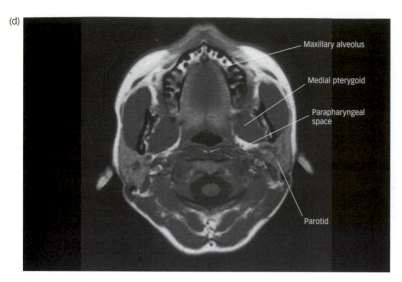

(d)

Maxillary alveolus

Medial pterygoid

Parapharyngeal space

Parotid

Fig. 10.14. *Continued*

The oropharynx extends from the nasopharynx to the upper border of the epiglottis inferiorly which, in turn, marks the upper limit of the laryngopharynx. The tonsils appear as symmetrical soft tissue densities on either side of the airway on CT. Both tonsils and adenoids are also well seen on MRI.

The laryngopharynx extends from the tip of the epiglottis to the esophagus at the level of the sixth cervical vertebra. The pharyngeal lumen is narrowest at its junction with the oesophagus where the cricopharyngeus forms the upper esophageal sphincter.

The fascial layers of the neck and the parapharyngeal space

Traditional anatomy describes several muscular triangles of the neck but cross-sectional imaging in contrast emphasizes the importance of the deep, fascia-lined spaces (Fig. 10.14) The fascia of the neck are divided into superficial and deep layers. The deep fascia define the deep spaces of the head and neck. These fascial layers form a barrier against the spread of inflammatory or neoplastic disease. The parapharyngeal space is easily recognized on both CT and MRI as a fatty triangle (Fig. 10.14) whose diagnostic importance is in the characteristic manner in which it is infiltrated, displaced or distorted by surrounding masses.

The larynx

The larynx forms the superior part of the lower respiratory tract and lies anterior to the laryngopharynx. Its cartilaginous skeleton (Fig. 10.15) contains the intrinsic muscles and the vocal folds. Laryngeal structures are well demonstrated by axial CT (Fig. 10.16) anteriorly lies the epiglottis, which arises from the posterior surface of the thyroid cartilage and is separated from the back of the tongue by paired depressions, the valleculae. The piriform fossae of the laryngopharynx lie between the laryngeal opening and the thyroid cartilage on each side.

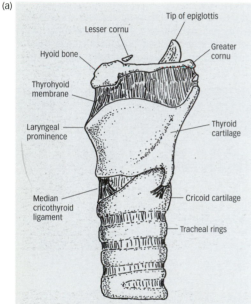

(a)

Tip of epiglottis

Lesser cornu

Hyoid bone

Greater cornu

Thyrohyoid membrane

Laryngeal prominence

Thyroid cartilage

Median cricothyroid ligament

Cricoid cartilage

Tracheal rings

Fig. 10.15(a),(b). **Diagram of the cartilaginous skeleton of the larynx: (a) external view, (b) cutaway view.**

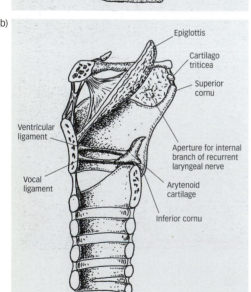

(b)

Epiglottis

Cartilago triticea

Superior cornu

Ventricular ligament

Aperture for internal branch of recurrent laryngeal nerve

Vocal ligament

Arytenoid cartilage

Inferior cornu

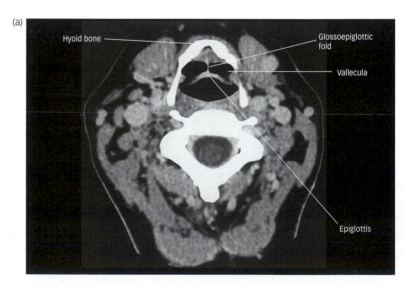

(a)

Hyoid bone

Glossoepiglottic fold

Vallecula

Epiglottis

Fig. 10.16(a)–(i). **Axial CT of the larynx from superior to inferior: (a) CT at level of hyoid bone showing tip of epiglottis and the valleculae anteriorly. Note the piriform fossae are below the level of the valleculae and are prominent laterally on (c)–(f). Note also the normally fatty preepiglottic and paraglottic spaces and that the fat is replaced by the glottic muscles at the level of the glottis.**

(b)

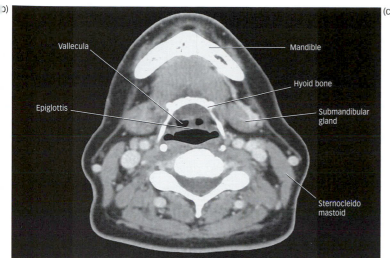

Vallecula

Mandible

Epiglottis

Hyoid bone

Submandibular gland

Sternocleido mastoid

(c)

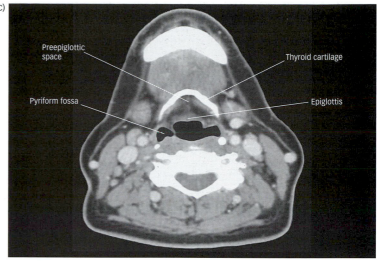

Preepiglottic space

Thyroid cartilage

Pyriform fossa

Epiglottis

(d)

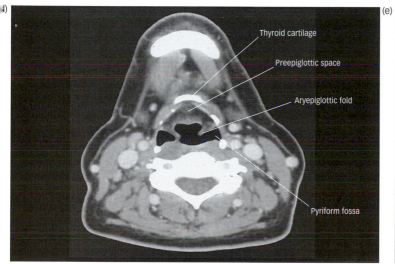

Thyroid cartilage

Preepiglottic space

Aryepiglottic fold

Pyriform fossa

(e)

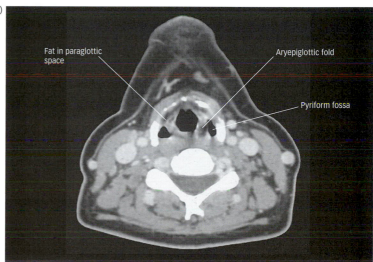

Fat in paraglottic space

Aryepiglottic fold

Pyriform fossa

(f)

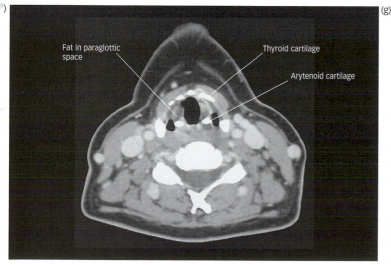

Fat in paraglottic space

Thyroid cartilage

Arytenoid cartilage

(g)

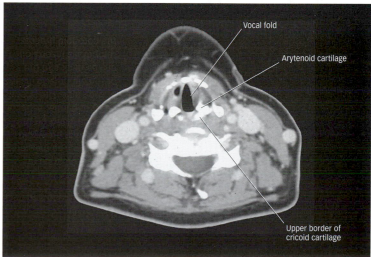

Vocal fold

Arytenoid cartilage

Upper border of cricoid cartilage

(h)

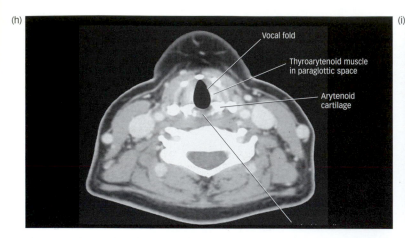

Vocal fold

Thyroarytenoid muscle in paraglottic space

Arytenoid cartilage

(i)

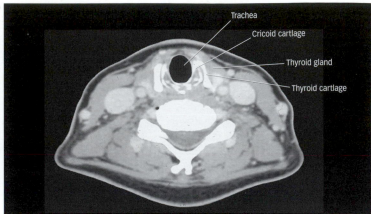

Trachea

Cricoid cartilage

Thyroid gland

Thyroid cartilage

Fig. 10.16(a)–(i). *Continued*

(a)

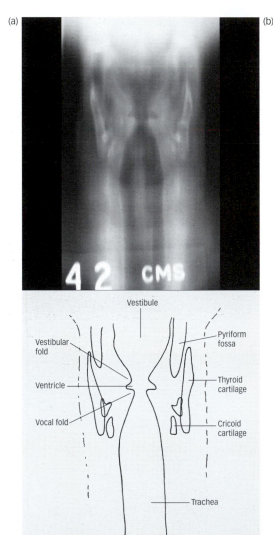

Vestibule

Vestibular fold

Ventricle

Vocal fold

Pyriform fossa

Thyroid cartilage

Cricoid cartilage

Trachea

(b)

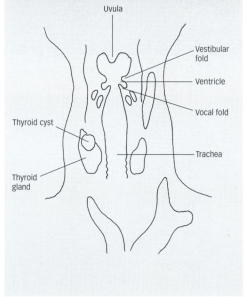

Fig. 10.17(a),(b). **Coronal views of the larynx: (a) soft tissue radiograph and (b) coronal MRI.**

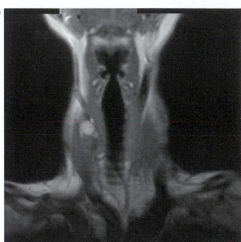

Uvula

Vestibular fold

Ventricle

Vocal fold

Trachea

Thyroid cyst

Thyroid gland

The inferior limit of the larynx is formed by the lower border of the cricoid cartilage, which articulates with the arytenoid cartilages. The arytenoids are capable of rotational and gliding movements, which alter the tension of the vocal cords.

The vocal cords are attached to the arytenoids, which are useful landmarks on CT to identify the vocal folds. The interior of the larynx is marked by the parallel bands of the true vocal cords inferiorly, and the vestibular folds or false cords superiorly. Between these is the slit-like cavity of the laryngeal ventricle. These structures are well seen in the coronal plane, on soft tissue radiographs, and on MRI scans (Fig. 10.17).

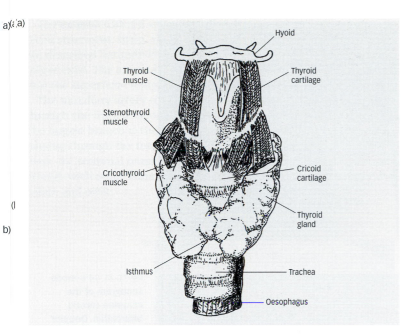

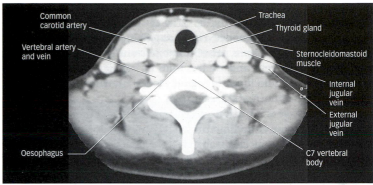

Fig. 10.19. **Contrast-enhanced CT of the neck at the level of the C7 vertebra. The thyroid gland shows intense enhancement. Posterolaterally lie the carotid sheaths. The vertebral vessels have not yet entered the foramen transversarium.**

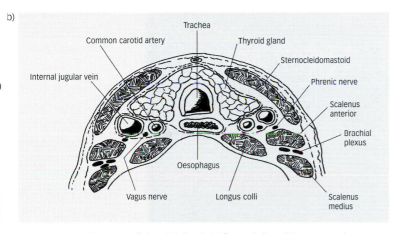

Fig. 10.18(a),(b). **Diagrams of thyroid gland: (a) frontal view (b) cross-section.**

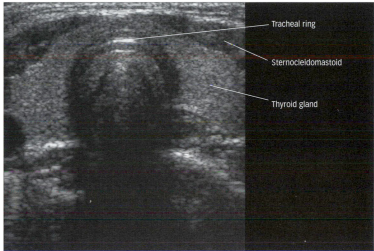

Fig. 10.20. **Ultrasound of the thyroid gland in transverse section. The lobes and isthmus of the thyroid gland with their normally homogeneous texture, lie on either side of the highly echoic tracheal rings. Superficial to the gland are the relatively hypoechoic sternocleidomastoid muscles.**

Thyroid and parathyroid glands

The thyroid gland extends on either side of the trachea linked by an isthmus (Fig. 10.18). The gland is enclosed by the deep cervical fascia and covered anteriorly by the strap muscles. Current imaging techniques show a relatively homogeneous texture. It is highly vascular however, and demonstrates intense contrast enhancement on CT and MRI (Fig. 10.19). Its superficial location makes the thyroid gland an ideal organ for ultrasound examination (Fig. 10.20).

Radionuclide imaging may be performed with [Tc^{99m}] pertechnetate, which is trapped by the thyroid in the same way as iodine and gives morphological information. It will reveal the presence of ectopic thyroid tissue (Fig. 10.21). Functional data can be obtained with the use of [^{23}I].

The normal parathyroid glands (four in number) are too small to be identified by imaging. Standard now for parathyroid tumour pick-up.

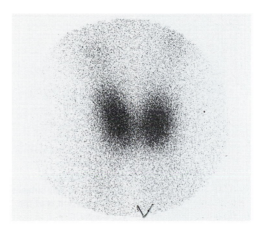

Fig. 10.21. **Thyroid scintigraphy.**

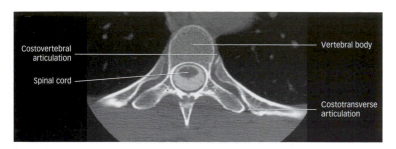

Fig. 11.13. **Axial CT myelogram, thoracic spine.**

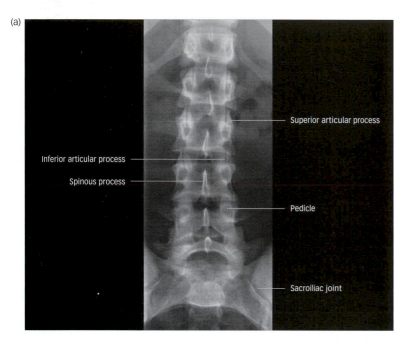

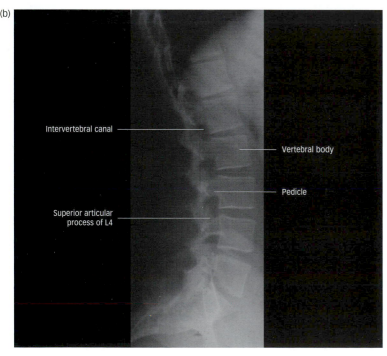

Fig. 11.14. **Lumbar spine radiographs: (a) anteroposterior, (b) lateral views.**

to the transverse process costotransverse joint (Fig. 11.13). Typically, therefore the ribs arise posteriorly between vertebrae. The first rib articulates only with T1 and similarly the tenth, eleventh, and twelfth ribs articulate only with T10, T11, and T12 vertebrae. At remaining levels, demifacets superior and inferior to the disk communicate with the head of the rib creating a costovertebral synovial joint. Therefore, the ribs arise posteriorly between vertebrae. In the thoracic region the canal is constant in size and circular in cross-section.

The lumbar vertebral column

There are five lumbar vertebrae, the third (L3) being the largest (Fig. 11.14). Lumbar vertebrae have square-shaped anterior vertebral bodies covered by fenestrated cartilage attached to the adjacent disks. Projecting posteriorly are bilateral pedicles composed of thick cortical bone connecting to lamina forming the spinal canal. The articular facets face each other in the sagittal plane (Fig. 11.15), and the transverse distance between the pedicles increases (the interpedicular distance) from L1 to L5. L5 is somewhat atypical with a wedge-shaped body, articulating inferiorly with the sacrum. Not infrequently, it may be fused, wholly or partly, with the body of the sacrum ("sacralization of L5"). Extending from the pedicles is a bony plate called the pars articularis from which extend the superior and inferior articular facets. The posterior superior articular facet of an inferiorly located vertebra connects to the posterior inferior facet of the superior vertebra above creating a diarthrodial synovial lined joint, surrounded by a fibrous capsule posterolaterally with absence of the joint capsule anteriorly, where the ligamentum flavum and synovial membrane are present, (Fig. 11.16).

The spinal cord

The spinal cord extends from the foramen magnum to the level of the first or second lumbar vertebrae. It is oval and elliptical in the cervical spine (Fig. 11.17), more rounded in the thoracic region (Fig. 11.18) always being wider in the transverse plane. A cleft anteriorly is referred to as the ventral median fissure and a small shallow sulcus is

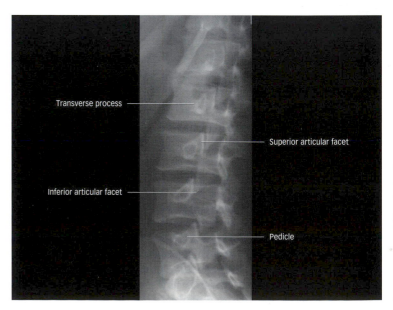

Fig. 11.15. **Lumbar spine radiograph, oblique projection.**

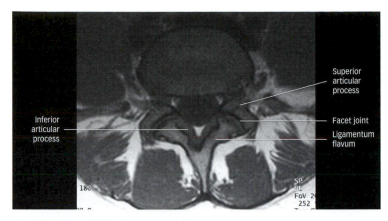

Fig. 11.16. **T1W axial MRI, lumbar vertebra.**

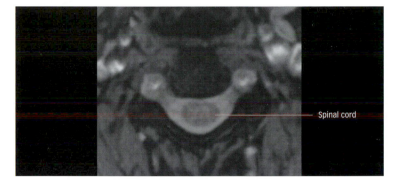

Fig. 11.17. **GRE axial MRI, cervical spine. Note that this sequence (gradient recalled echo) demonstrates gray matter within the spinal cord.**

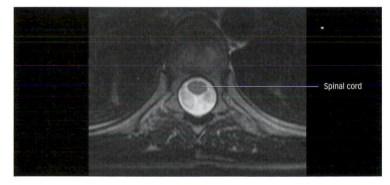

Fig. 11.18. **T2W axial MRI, thoracic spine.**

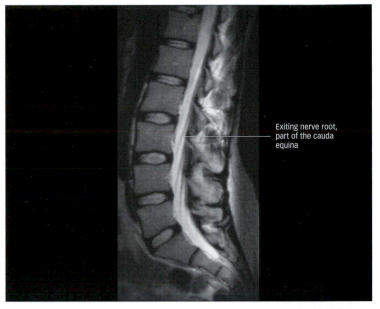

Fig. 11.19. **T2W sagittal MRI, lumbar spine showing the cauda equina.**

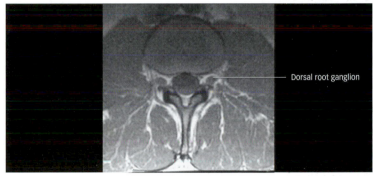

Fig. 11.20. **T1W axial image, lumbar vertebra.**

noted posteriorly. In cross-section the cord has central gray matter shaped like a butterfly H-shaped pattern surrounded by white matter.

The lower end of the spinal cord tapers to form the conus medullaris and from the conus the thin filum terminale extends to the coccyx.

The caliber of the spinal cord increases in two regions as the cervical (C5–T1 segments) and lumbar (L2–S3 segments) expansions concerned with the arms and legs, respectively.

The spinal nerves

Since the spinal cord is shorter than the vertebral column, the spinal nerves take a progressively oblique course caudally to emerge through the intervertebral canals. Below the termination of the spinal cord, the nerve roots in the lumbar region pass almost vertically down to form the cauda equina (horse's tail) (Fig. 11.19).

There are 31 pairs of spinal nerves: 8 cervical, 12 thoracic and 5 lumbar. Each spinal nerve is formed from a dorsal (posterior) sensory root and a ventral (anterior) motor root emerging from the spinal cord. The ventral roots contain axons of the neurons in the spinal gray matter. The neurons of the dorsal roots are found in the ganglion borne by each dorsal root. The ganglion is usually situated in the intervertebral canal (Fig. 11.20) and distal to this ventral and dorsal roots merge to form the spinal nerve (Fig. 11.2a). C1 root exits between the occiput and C1 vertebra. Each cervical nerve root therefore exits above the correspondingly numbered vertebra. C8 root exits between C7 and T1 vertebrae. Because of this, thoracic nerve roots exit below the correspondingly numbered thoracic vertebra.

In the lumbar spine each root leaves the spinal canal laterally below the pedicle of the corresponding vertebra and above the disk.

Meninges

The spinal and cranial meningeal sheaths are continuous. The spinal dural sac extends from the posterior cranial fossa to the second sacral segment. It surrounds the spinal cord, nerve roots and cerebrospinal fluid (CSF).

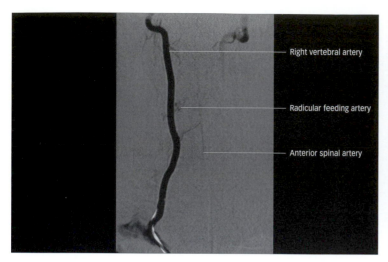

Fig. 11.21. **Vertebral angiogram showing the anterior spinal artery and radicular arteries.**

- Right vertebral artery
- Radicular feeding artery
- Anterior spinal artery

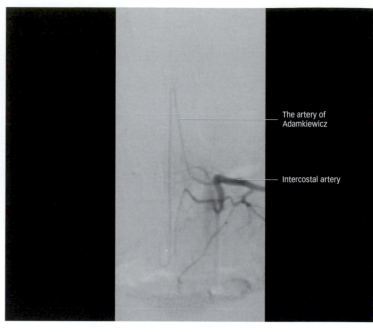

- The artery of Adamkiewicz
- Intercostal artery

Fig. 11.22. **The artery of Adamkiewicz arising from the left intercostal artery at T9 level.**

Within the dura is the avascular arachnoid and the pia mater, the second component of the leptomeninges, forms a layer over the spinal cord. Between the two is the subarachnoid space, which contains cerebrospinal fluid.

The blood supply to the spinal cord

The cervical spinal cord blood supply is from the anterior spinal artery and paired posterior spinal arteries. The anterior spinal artery is formed superiorly from branches that extend inferiorly from both of the vertebral arteries (Fig. 11.21). It supplies the anterior two-thirds of the cord. This critical area includes the corticospinal and spinothalamic tracts as well as the central gray matter anterior column.

The posterior spinal arteries, which also arise from the vertebral arteries, supply the posterior one-third of the cord, including the posterior columns and central gray matter posterior horn.

The spinal arteries, running the length of the cord, also receive numerous contributions from various cervical arteries and from the segmental thoracic intercostal and lumbar arteries. These feeding vessels extend through the intervertebral canals and bifurcate into anterior and posterior vessels extending along the dorsal and ventral nerve roots. One very important major contribution comes from the Artery of Adamkiewicz, which usually arises from the left side and/or the intercostals arteries at the T-9 to T-12 vertebral levels. This vessel comes into the spinal canal with nerve roots and has a classic "hairpin loop" (Fig. 11.22). This vessel supplies the anterior spinal cord in the thoracolumbar region via a large descending vessel which anastamoses with the posterior spinal arteries at the conus. Draining veins leave the spinal cord through the intervertebral canals to join an extensive interconnecting plexus of veins in the epidural space.

Section 5 | The limbs

Chapter 12 | The upper limb

ALEX M. BARNACLE
and ADAM W. M. MITCHELL

The skeletal anatomy of the upper limb is well demonstrated on conventional plain radiographs, which are quick and simple to acquire and have better spatial resolution than computed tomography (CT) or magnetic resonance imaging (MRI). Radiographs are usually acquired in two planes, at 90 degrees to one another, to overcome issues such as foreshortening and overlying bony structures. When imaging complex joints such as the shoulder, supplementary views may also be required.

In complex orthopedic or trauma cases, 3-D image reconstructions of CT examinations provide excellent visualization of regions of abnormal skeletal development or complex fractures. MRI is more often applied in the assessment of soft tissues, including the joints, the neurovascular structures, especially the brachial plexus, and the bone marrow. Ultrasound (US) is used increasingly commonly in the evaluation of the superficial soft tissue structures, such as the tendons of the rotator cuff within the shoulder and the tendons of the wrist.

Arthrography involves the injection of a contrast agent such as air or iodinated contrast medium into a joint space to allow visualization of the joint, its capsule and articular surfaces under fluoroscopy. This technique has been largely superseded by other imaging modalities such as MRI, although arthrography combined with MR or CT, where gadolinium or iodinated contrast medium is instilled into the joint prior to imaging, gives exquisite detail of the joint spaces and any disruption of the joint capsule or supporting structures.

Angiography and venography are used to assess arterial and venous anatomy for reasons such as the placement of central venous catheters, planning the formation and maintenance of arteriovenous fistulas and the management of arterial trauma. This can be performed via traditional catheter angiography techniques or by digitally reconstructing the vascular detail from a contrast medium enhanced CT or magnetic resonance (MR) examination

In most musculoskeletal cases, more than one imaging modality is required to acquire the breadth of radiological information necessary to make a full and accurate diagnosis.

The shoulder and upper arm

The shoulder girdle
The shoulder girdle connects the upper limb to the axial skeleton, allowing movement at both the shoulder joint and the scapulothoracic joint (Fig. 12.1). The weight of the arm is transmitted to the trunk primarily via the clavicle.

The scapula
The scapula overlies the posterolateral aspect of the chest wall, its inner surface closely applied to the posterior aspects of the second to

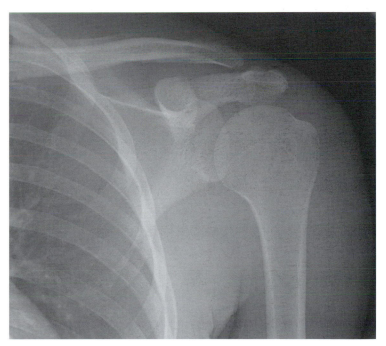

Fig. 12.1. **Anteroposterior radiograph of the left shoulder.**

Applied Radiological Anatomy for Medical Students. Paul Butler, Adam Mitchell, and Harold Ellis (eds.) Published by Cambridge University Press. © P. Butler, A. Mitchell, and H. Ellis 2007.

seventh ribs. The anterior and posterior surfaces of the scapula give attachment to many of the muscles of the rotator cuff. The rotator cuff is the term used to describe the tendons of the four smaller muscles surrounding the shoulder joint; the tendons are intimately related to the capsule of the shoulder joint (Fig. 12.2). Subscapularis attaches to the convex costal surface of the scapula and inserts onto the lesser tubercle of the humerus. Supraspinatus arises from the supraspinous fossa of the posterior aspect of the scapula and inserts onto the greater tubercle of the humerus. Adjacent to this, infraspinatus arises from the infraspinous fossa and also attaches to the greater tubercle. The supraspinous and infraspinous fossae communicate laterally around the base of the spine of the scapula. Teres minor arises from the lateral margin of the scapula and inserts inferiorly onto the greater tubercle of the humerus.

Laterally, the angle of the scapula forms the articular surface of the bone, known as the glenoid fossa; this articulates with the humeral head. The bony tubercles above and below the glenoid fossa give attachment to the long heads of biceps and triceps respectively. The projection known as the acromion is formed by the flattened lateral extension of the spine of the scapula. It articulates with the lateral end of the clavicle and overlies the shoulder joint, providing some protection for both the joint and the overlying supraspinatus tendon of the rotator cuff. Medial to the acromion, the coracoid process of the scapula projects anteriorly, giving attachment to the short head of biceps, pectoralis minor, and coracobrachialis, and to the coracoclavicular ligament. Latissimus dorsi, teres major, and serratus anterior attach to the inferior angle of the body of the scapula. The acromion and the spine of the scapula give attachment to larger muscles of the shoulder girdle, trapezius, and deltoid.

The clavicle

The clavicle is an S-shaped bone that develops from a mesenchymal or membranous origin and is the first bone in the body to ossify. It is unusual in that it does not contain a medullary cavity. The clavicle articulates with the manubrium of the sternum and the first costal cartilage medially, forming the sternoclavicular joint. The costoclavicular ligament arises from the inferior surface of the medial clavicle and inserts onto the upper surface of the first costal cartilage and the first rib. Laterally, the clavicle articulates with the acromion of the scapula, the coracoclavicular ligament arising from the inferior surface of the clavicle just medial to this joint. The large muscles of the shoulder girdle gain some of their attachments from the clavicle: pectoralis major, deltoid, sternocleidomastoid and trapezius.

The clavicle transmits part of the weight of the upper limb to the trunk and, with the scapula, allows the arm to swing clear of the trunk.

The sternoclavicular joint

The fibrocartilaginous sternoclavicular joint is formed by the articulation of the manubrium sternum and the first costal cartilage with the medial aspect of the clavicle. The strong fibrous costoclavicular ligament arises from the inferior surface of the clavicle just lateral to the sternoclavicular joint, attaching to the superior aspect of the first rib and stabilizing the joint. Further stability is afforded by the

(a)
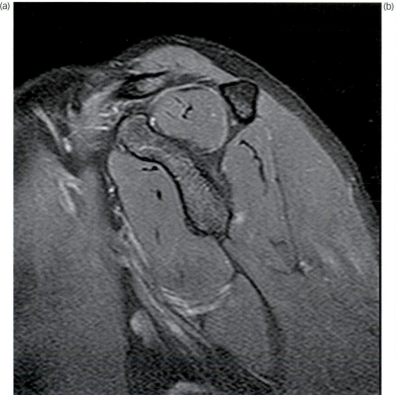
(b)
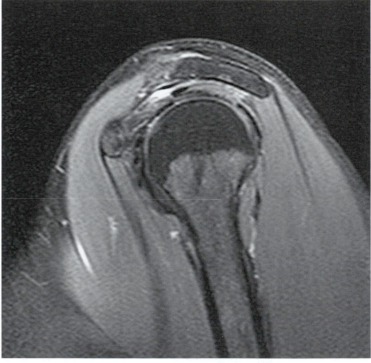

Fig. 12.2. **T2 weighted MR images acquired in the sagittal plane (lateral view): (a) image through the body of the scapula, the coracoid process and acromion. The muscles of the rotator cuff surround the body of the scapula; (b) More lateral image through the humeral head showing the tendons of the rotator cuff before their insertion onto the humerus.**

interclavicular ligament, which lies within the suprasternal notch, and focal thickening of the joint capsule known as the anterior and posterior sternoclavicular ligaments. Each joint contains a fibrocartilagenous disk dividing the joint into medial and lateral synovial compartments.

The joint is capable of small movements, which are associated with movement at the acromioclavicular joint and which act to increase the range of movement of the whole upper limb. Movements at the sternoclavicular joint include elevation and depression, horizontal forward and backward movement, circumduction, and axial rotation.

The acromioclavicular joint

The acromioclavicular joint is a complex synovial joint between the lateral border of the clavicle and the medial aspect of the acromion of the scapula. The joint contains an incomplete fibrocartilaginous disk and is surrounded by a weak synovial joint capsule. Accessory ligaments comprise the aromioclavicular ligament, a fibrous band that overlies the superior surface of the joint, and the coracoclavicular ligament that extends from the inferior surface of the clavicle to the superior surface of the coracoid process, providing a strong attachment of the clavicle to the scapula and lending stability to the joint. Disruption of the ligaments or the joint capsule itself will result in widening of the joint space, and the clavicle will override the acromion.

The supraspinatus tendon runs immediately below the acromioclavicular joint. Any degenerative disease in the joint may cause irregularity of the under surface of the joint, which in turn causes wear and tear of the tendon, and loss of the normal tendon thickness. When assessing plain radiographs of the shoulder, observe the soft tissues inferior to the acromioclavicular joint for narrowing of the distance between it and the humeral head and for calcification within the supraspinatus tendon. Ultrasound examination of the shoulder provides useful "real-time" imaging of the rotator cuff (Fig. 12.3). Changes in the reflectivity of the tendons and the surface of the bony contours are suggestive of inflammatory or degenerative change. Dynamic information can also be gained by imaging the shoulder in different positions and during movement.

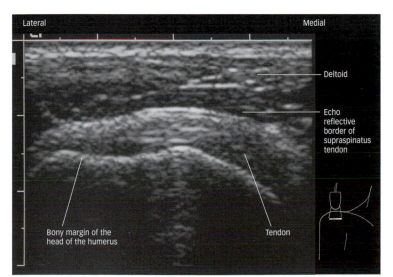

Fig. 12.3. **Ultrasound image of the shoulder, showing the hyperechoic superior border of the supraspinatus tendon. The contour of the bony surface of the humeral head remains smooth.**

The humerus

The hemispherical head of the humerus articulates with the glenoid fossa of the scapula. The anatomical neck of the humerus is formed by the boundary of the joint capsule. The surgical neck is the term used for the slightly narrowed junction between the head of the humerus and its shaft, because of the tendency of the humerus to fracture at this point. The lateral aspect of the humeral head forms two prominent tubercles, known as the greater and lesser tuberosities or tubercles, which are separated by the intertubercular or bicipital groove. The greater tuberosity lies posterior to the lesser tuberosity. Many of the tendons of the rotator cuff insert onto the humeral tubercles: supraspinatus, infraspinatus, and teres minor attach to the greater tuberosity and subscapularis to the lesser tuberosity. The long head of biceps lies within a vertical channel known as the bicipital groove.

A spiral groove along the posterior aspect of the shaft of the humerus accommodates the radial nerve. Deltoid inserts onto a small protrusion on the lateral aspect of the shaft known as the deltoid tuberosity, triceps attaches posteriorly and brachialis anteriorly. The neurovascular bundle of the median nerve, brachial artery, and basilic vein lies more superficially, medial to the humerus.

At the elbow, the humerus expands and flattens to form the medial and lateral supracondylar ridges and the medial and lateral epicondyles, from which the common flexor and extensor origins, respectively, arise. The lateral rounded capitellum and the medial trochlea form the articular surfaces of the humerus at the elbow. The fat-filled olecranon fossa posteriorly accommodates the olecranon process of the ulna during elbow flexion, and a similar fossa anteriorly accommodates the head of the radius.

The glenohumeral joint

The glenohumeral or shoulder joint is a synovial ball and socket joint. The shallow glenoid fossa is deepened by the glenoid labrum, a circumferential outer fibrocartilaginous ring (Fig. 12.4). Even with the labrum present, the articular surface of the glenoid remains less than one-third of the surface area of the humeral head. The joint capsule attaches to the glenoid labrum and inserts into the articular margin of the humeral head, except inferiorly where it extends on to the medial aspect of the humeral neck. The anterior portion of the joint capsule is strengthened by the three glenohumeral ligaments surrounding the shoulder joint. The capsule is lax inferiorly, as demonstrated by arthrography (Fig. 12.5). The tendon of the long head of biceps runs through the joint capsule, enclosed by the synovial membrane of the capsule, and can therefore be involved in diseases of the joint. The transverse humeral ligament is an accessory ligament of the shoulder joint; it bridges the intertubercular groove between the greater and lesser tuberosities, holding the long tendon of biceps in place.

The movements of the shoulder joint are:

- *Flexion*: clavicular head of pectoralis major, anterior fibers of deltoid, coracobrachialis
- *Extension*: posterior fibers of deltoid, reinforced in the flexed position by latissimus dorsi, pectoralis major, teres major
- *Abduction*: initiated by supraspinatus, continued by deltoid
- *Adduction*: pectoralis major, latissimus dorsi, subscapularis, teres major
- *Medial rotation*: pectoralis major, anterior fibres of deltoid, latissimus dorsi, teres major, subscapularis
- *Lateral rotation*: posterior fibres of deltoid, teres minor, infraspinatus.

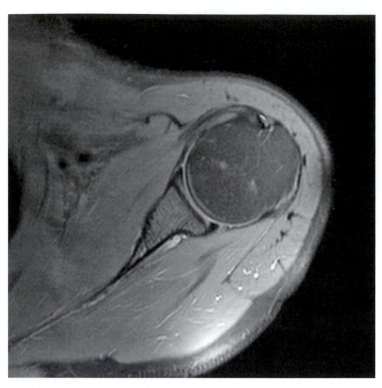

Fig. 12.4. **T2 weighted axial MR image at the level of the head of the humerus, showing the low signal labrum projecting from the margins of the glenoid and a sliver of high signal synovial fluid within the joint.**

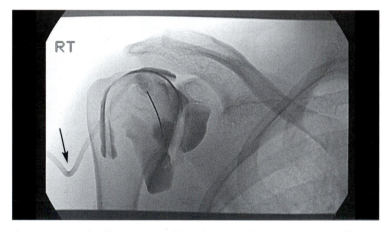

Fig. 12.5. **Conventional arthrogram of the shoulder. Iodinated contrast medium has been instilled into the joint through a butterfly cannula, which is seen overlying the image (arrow). Contrast fills the joint capsule and outlines the tendon of the long head of biceps.**

As mentioned above, movement of the shoulder girdle increases the range of movement of the shoulder. Note that flexion/extension at the shoulder joint does not occur in a true anteroposterior plane; in flexion, the upper arm moves anteriorly and medially, so that anatomical flexion of the shoulder involves a degree of abduction.

Musculature of the shoulder

Pectoralis major arises from the anterior chest wall structures, which comprise the sternum, the upper six costal cartilages, the anterior surface of the clavicle, and the aponeurosis of external oblique. It inserts on to the lateral lip of the humeral intertubercular groove.

Pectoralis minor lies deep to pectoralis major, arising medially from the anterior surfaces of the third, fourth, and fifth ribs and inserting onto the coracoid process of the scapula.

Serratus anterior arises from the lateral aspects of the upper eight ribs, forming the medial wall of the axilla. It attaches to the costal surface of medial border of the scapula.

Trapezius is a broad, flat, superficial muscle arising from the nuchal line of the occiput, the ligamentum nuchae, the thoracic vertebral spines, and the supraspinous ligaments. It inserts onto the lateral aspect of the clavicle, the acromion, and the scapula spine. Latissimus dorsi has an extensive origin, including the spines and supraspinous ligaments of the lower six thoracic vertebrae, the thoracolumbar fascia of the back, the posterior part of the iliac crest, and the lower four ribs. It forms a strap-like tendon that inserts on to the floor of the intertubercular groove of the humerus.

Levator scapulae and the major and minor rhomboids lie deep to trapezius, running from the thoracic vertebrae to the medial border of the scapula.

Deltoid arises from the lateral third of the clavicle, the acromion, and the scapular spine, inserting on to the deltoid tuberosity of the body of the humerus.

Teres major forms part of the posterior axillary wall, arising from the lateral border and angle of the scapula and inserting onto the medial lip of the intertubercular groove of the humerus.

The muscles of the rotator cuff have been covered in the scapula section.

Bursae of the shoulder

A bursa is a sac lined with a synovial membrane, which secretes lubricating synovial fluid. Bursas usually occur around joints and serve to reduce friction at sites where tendons or ligaments rub across bony structures.

The glenohumeral joint is surrounded by several bursae. The most clinically significant of these is the large subacromial–subdeltoid bursa, which lies between the supraspinatus and the inferior surface of the coracoacromial arch. This bursa does not communicate with the joint capsule unless the supraspinatus tendon is ruptured. Spill of contrast medium into the bursa during joint arthrography therefore implies disruption of the supraspinatus muscle or tendon.

Imaging of the shoulder

The standard plain radiographic views of the shoulder are the anteroposterior (Fig. 12.1) and axial projections (Fig. 12.6). The axial view allows assessment of the congruity of the glenohumeral joint. In suspected shoulder dislocation, the trans-scapular view provides information on the relationship of the humeral head to the glenoid fossa, which is projected behind the humeral head (Fig. 12.7). The Striker's view is acquired with the beam angled through the axilla to provide anatomical detail of the posterior aspect of the humeral head, which is obscured on the axial view and may be damaged in cases of recurrent dislocation (Fig. 12.8).

The fibrocartilaginous components of the shoulder joint and its surrounding tendons are well demonstrated on MR. Information regarding the joint capsule, the bony configuration of the humeral head, and the integrity of the labrum can be acquired by instilling arthrographic contrast medium into the joint capsule. Arthrography can be performed using air or iodinated contrast medium, and then acquiring

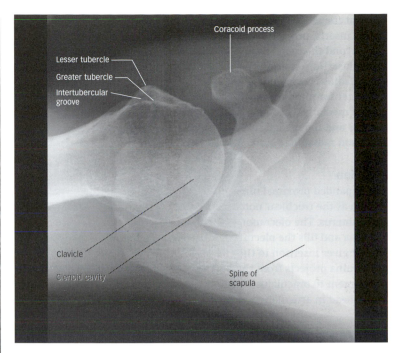

Fig. 12.6. **Axial radiograph of the shoulder.**

- Coracoid process
- Lesser tubercle
- Greater tubercle
- Intertubercular groove
- Clavicle
- Glenoid cavity
- Spine of scapula

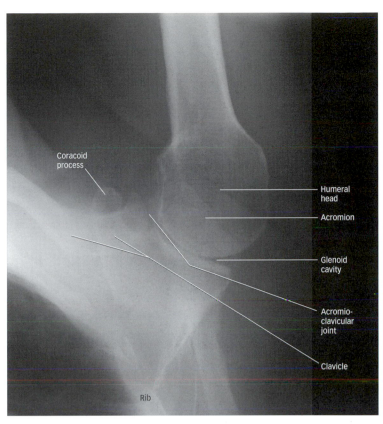

Fig. 12.8. **Striker's view of the shoulder. This view clearly demonstrates the posterior aspect of the humeral head.**

- Coracoid process
- Humeral head
- Acromion
- Glenoid cavity
- Acromio-clavicular joint
- Clavicle
- Rib

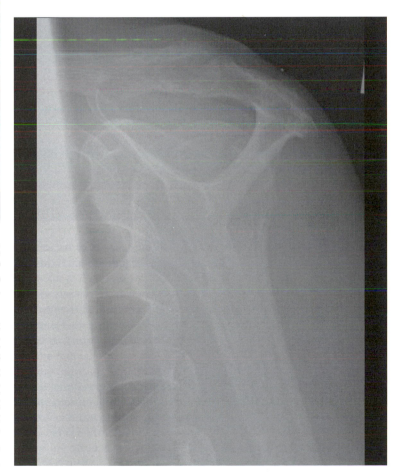

Fig. 12.7. **Trans-scapular radiograph of the shoulder. The body of the scapula is projected behind the shaft of the humerus and the glenoid fossa is seen en face.**

radiographs to demonstrate the extent of the joint capsule (see Fig. 12.5). Alternatively, MR contrast agents such as gadolinium can be instilled prior to MR examination of the shoulder, allowing very detailed imaging of the labrum and the articular surface (Fig. 12.9).

The axilla

The axilla lies between the lateral chest wall and the upper arm. The fat-filled pyramidal space contains the axillary artery and vein, cords and terminal branches of the brachial plexus, the coracobracialis and biceps muscles, and the axillary lymph nodes. The apex of the space is formed by the first rib and the middle third of the clavicle. The medial wall of the axilla is made up of the lateral aspects of the upper four ribs and their accompanying intercostal muscles and fascia, and serratus anterior. The anterior wall is bounded by pectoralis major and minor, the posterior wall by subscapularis, latissimus dorsi and teres major, and the lateral wall by the intertubercular groove of the humerus onto which the muscles of the anterior and posterior walls insert. The base of the axilla is formed by skin and superficial fascia. This allows an excellent window for ultrasound examination of the axilla, which is useful in the assessment of soft tissue pathology such as lymphadenopathy. The structures of the axilla are also well demonstrated on MRI.

The musculature of the arm

The musculature of the upper arm is divided into two compartments by the medial and lateral intermuscular septa, which extend from the humerus to fuse with the deep fascia of the arm. The anterior component contains the flexor muscles: the biceps, coracobrachialis and

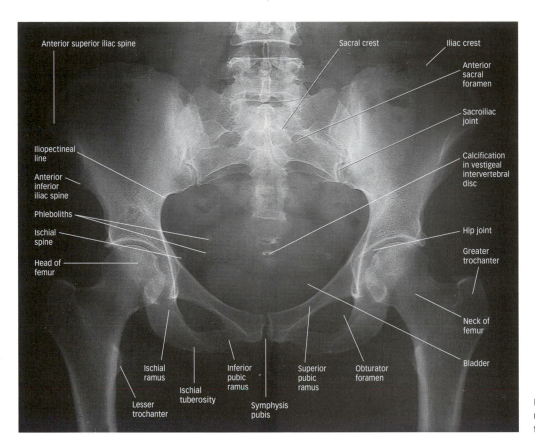

Fig. 13.1. **Frontal radiograph of an adult female pelvis.**

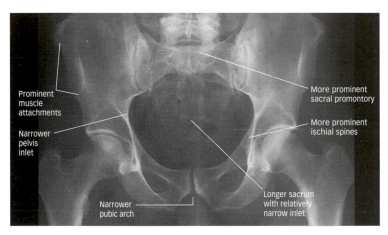

Fig. 13.2. **Frontal radiograph of an adult male pelvis. Note the differences between this radiograph and that of the female pelvis illustrated in Fig. 13.1.**

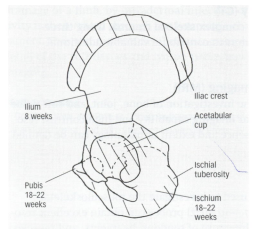

Fig. 13.3. **Ossification of the bones of the pelvis. The secondary centres (hatched) start to ossify at puberty and fuse at 20–25 years.**

promontory, ilio-pectineal lines, and symphysis pubis. The pelvic outlet is bounded by the coccyx posteriorly, the ischial tuberosities laterally, and the inferior pubic arch anteriorly.

The sacroiliac joints

These are synovial joints between the auricular surfaces of the sacrum and iliac bones. The iliac surface is covered with hyaline cartilage, the sacral surface by fibrocartilage. A small amount of rotatory movement occurs at the joint, which is increased in pregnancy and childbearing. The joint is strengthened by the ventral and dorsal sacroiliac ligaments and particularly by the interosseous sacroiliac ligament which occupies the area immediately above and behind the joint.

Three accessory ligaments also contribute to the stability of the posterior part of the pelvic ring.

The symphysis pubis

This is a secondary cartilaginous joint, consisting of both hyaline and fibrocartilage. (Primary cartilaginous joints contain only hyaline cartilage.) Each articular surface is covered with a layer of hyaline cartilage enclosing a fibrocartilaginous disk. The whole joint is covered by dense ligaments. Virtually no movement is possible at the joint.

There are some gender differences in the appearance of the pelvis visible on plain radiographs (Fig. 13.2).

Ossification of the pelvis is demonstrated in Fig. 13.3.

The hip joint

This is a synovial articulation of the "ball and socket" type between the head of the femur and the acetabulum. The articular cartilage is thickest and broadest superiorly where the weight is borne. The fovea capitis, where the ligament of the head (ligamentum teres) is attached, is not covered in cartilage. The articular surface of the acetabulum is deficient inferiorly over the acetabular notch and centrally where the floor of the acetabulum is filled with a fiberofatty pad. The fibrocartilaginous acetabular labrum serves to deepen the articular cup. It bridges the acetabular notch as the transverse acetabular ligament. The fibrous capsule is attached around the rim of the acetabulum and inferiorly to the transverse acetabular ligament. It is reinforced by three ligaments (Fig. 13.4). Its femoral attachments are to the base of the neck and to the inter-trochanteric line.

The capsular retinaculum is made up of fibers that are reflected proximally along the neck. It carries an important part of the blood supply to the femoral head and neck.

The synovium arises from the margins of the articular cartilage of the femoral neck and covers the intracapsular femoral neck, the inner surface of the capsule, the acetabular labrum, the fibrofatty pad filling in the floor of the acetabulum and is reflected as a tube sheathing the ligamentum teres. It may communicate with a bursa beneath the tendon of psoas major through a deficiency in the fibrous capsule and iliofemoral ligament.

The movements of the hip joint are

- *flexion*: iliacus, psoas major, pectineus, rectus femoris, and sartorius;
- *extension*: gluteus maximus and the hamstrings;
- *abduction*: gluteus medius and minimus, tensor fascia lata, and sartorius;
- *adduction*: adductor longus, brevis and magnus, pectineus, and gracilis;
- *medial rotation*: anterior fibers of gluteus medius and minimus, tensor fascia lata;
- *lateral rotation*: obturator muscles, gemelli, quadratus femoris, piriformis, gluteus maximus, and sartorius.

A brief outline of the attachment of the most important muscles of the lower limb is given below to supplement the images and diagrams of the cross-sectional anatomy (Fig. 13.5).

Gluteus maximus arises from the superior part of the posterior surface of the ilium including the crest, the side of the sacrum, coccyx, and sacrotuberous ligament. The majority of the muscle converges as a tendinous sheet to merge with the iliotibial tract. The deeper fibers attach to the gluteal tuberosity of the femur. Gluteus medius arises deep to, and below, gluteus maximus and attaches to the lateral aspect of the greater trochanter. Gluteus minimus arises below, and deep to, gluteus medius and is completely covered by it. It is attached to the anterior surface of the greater trochanter.

Piriformis arises from the front of the sacrum and from the gluteal surface of the ilium. It passes out of the pelvis through the greater sciatic foramen and inserts on the upper border of the greater trochanter.

Obturator internus arises from the pelvic surface of the medial part of the obturator membrane and the surrounding bone and passes through the lesser sciatic foramen. Its tendon receives the fibers of the gemelli muscles and inserts at the medial surface of the greater trochanter.

Obturator externus takes its origin from the outer surface of the obturator membrane and the surrounding bone and passes below the hip joint to insert at the base of the medial surface of the greater trochanter.

Plain radiography relies mainly on the anteroposterior (AP) view (Fig. 13.6), and several landmarks should be identified. Shenton's line is a smooth curve running from the medial aspect of the femoral neck to the superior border of the obturator foramen. The iliopectineal line and ilio-ischial lines should also be smooth symmetrical arcs.

The posterior and anterior rims of the acetabulum and the acetabular "teardrop" are also illustrated. Kohler's "teardrop distance" should be less than 11 mm, and there should not be a difference of more than 2 mm between the two sides.

Imaging of the pelvis and hips

A lateral film is often required to rule out subtle fractures of the femoral neck (Fig. 13.6). A "frog" lateral is sometimes obtained using

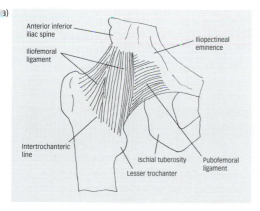
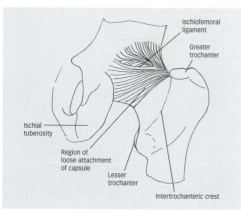

Fig. 13.4. **The ligaments of the right hip joint, (a) anterior, (b) posterior.**

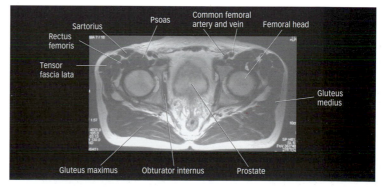

Fig. 13.5. **Proton density axial MRI: the hip joints**

(a)

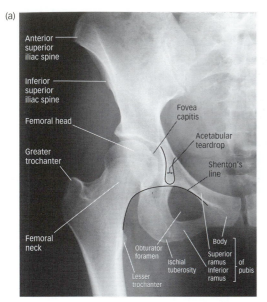

Anterior
superior
iliac spine

Inferior
superior
iliac spine

Femoral head

Greater
trochanter

Femoral
neck

Fovea
capitis

Acetabular
teardrop

Shenton's
line

Obturator
foramen

Ischial
tuberosity

Lesser
trochanter

Body

Superior
ramus
Inferior
ramus

of
pubis

(b)

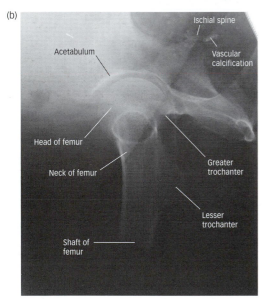

Acetabulum

Head of femur

Neck of femur

Shaft of
femur

Ischial spine

Vascular
calcification

Greater
trochanter

Lesser
trochanter

Fig. 13.6. **AP and lateral Radiographs of the right hip, (a) anteroposterior, (b) lateral.**

an AP radiograph with the hip abducted and externally rotated so that the knee is lying nearly on the table top. The frog lateral is particularly useful in assessing the femoral capital epiphyses in children and comparing one side with the other. Other views occasionally used include oblique (Judet's) views of the acetabulum and pelvic inlet and outlet views in cases of pelvic trauma.

Ultrasound is able to detect small amounts of fluid within the joint; the anterior surface of the femoral neck within the joint capsule is accessible to high resolution scanning.

CT is particularly useful in the evaluation of complex bony injuries of the pelvis, sacro-iliac joints and for identifying bony fragments in the acetabulum.

MRI is increasingly being used to make the early diagnosis of avascular necrosis of the hip, a condition for which MR has a high sensitivity and specificity. It is also able to characterize the soft tissues, ligaments, and the acetabular labrum.

Arthrography is rarely necessary, although it is often helpful if combined with manual or digital subtraction techniques in the assessment

of hip prostheses, especially in the context of possible loosening. Arthrography also increases the accuracy of MR in detecting labral tears and small articular cartilage defects.

Pelvimetry

It is occasionally necessary to assess the female pelvis radiologically to assess the likelihood of difficulties in labor.

MRI should be used if available as it imparts no radiation dose. CT pelvimetry is more commonly used, especially outside pregnancy, and is performed using a lateral scout view and measuring the inlet and outlet diameters in the sagittal plane.

The most important measurement is the AP inlet or conjugate diameter, which is the smallest AP diameter between the posterior margin of the symphysis pubis and the anterior aspect of the sacrum, (Fig. 13.7). The normal value varies between 11.0 and 12.5 cm. Values of less than 10.5 cm indicate increasing likelihood of cephalopelvic disproportion.

The thigh

The femur

The femur (Fig. 13.8), consists of a shaft, a neck, and a head, which articulates with the acetabulum. The patella is a flattened sesamoid bone within the quadriceps tendon. Ossification is shown in Fig. 13.9.

The muscles of the thigh (Fig. 13.10)
Anterior femoral muscles

Tensor fascia lata arises from the anterior superior iliac spine (ASIS) and is inserted into the iliotibial tract, a strong thickened band of the deep fascia of the lateral aspect of the thigh (fascia lata), which is attached distally to Gerdy's tubercle on the antero-lateral condyle of the tibia.

Sartorius is a narrow strap muscle arising from the ASIS, which descends diagonally across the front of the thigh to the medial aspect of the knee, where it inserts on the medial tibial condyle.

Quadriceps femoris is made up of four components. Rectus femoris arises by a straight head from the anterior inferior iliac spine (AIIS) and a reflected head from the superior margin of the acetabulum and the capsule of the hip joint. Its tendon inserts into the superior border of the patella. Vastus intermedius arises from the anterior surface of the femoral shaft and inserts into the superior border of the patella deep to the tendon of rectus femoris. Vastus lateralis arises from the greater trochanter and the upper part of the linea aspera. Its distal tendon inserts into the outer border of the patella and blends with the iliotibial tract. Vastus medialis arises from the lower part of the greater trochanter and the anterior surface of the femur. Its tendon inserts into the medial side of the patella. The patellar retinacula are expansions of the distal tendons of vastus medialis and lateralis.

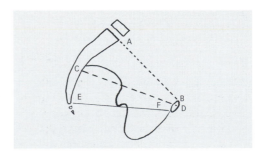

Fig. 13.7. **Measurements obtained during CT. AB = conjugate inlet diameter; EF = conjugate outlet diameter pelvimetry.**

(a)

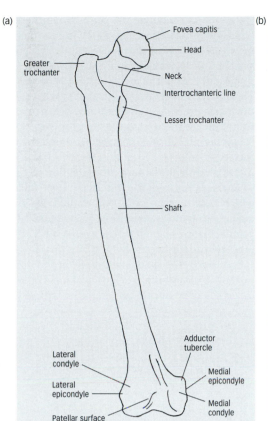

(b)

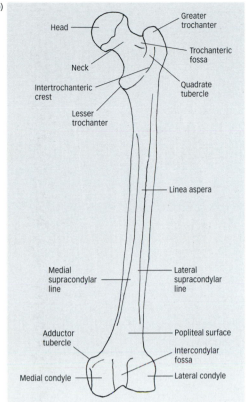

Fig. 13.8. **The right femur, (a) anterior, (b) posterior.**

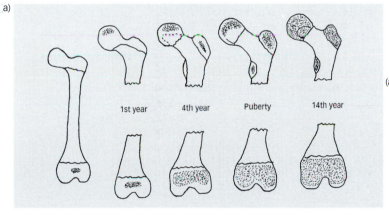

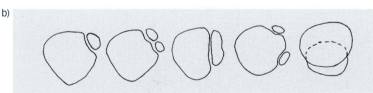

Fig. 13.9. **(a) Ossification of femur. The secondary centres fuse with the shaft at 18–20 years; (b) bipartite and multipartite patellae.**

The adductor muscles

Gracilis arises from the body and inferior ramus of the pubis and passes down the medial aspect of the thigh over the medial femoral condyle to insert into the medial surface of the tibia below the condyle. Pectineus is a flat, quadrilateral muscle arising from the pubis; it passes posterolaterally to insert between the lesser

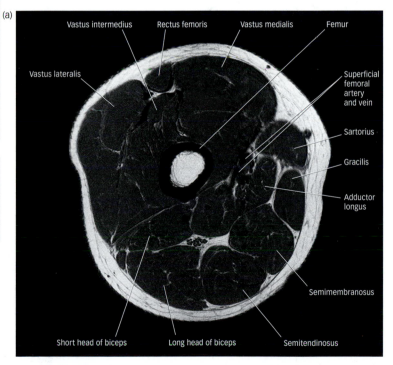

Fig. 13.10. **IW MRI of the right thigh: (a) axial scan through mid-thigh and (b) coronal image.**

(b)

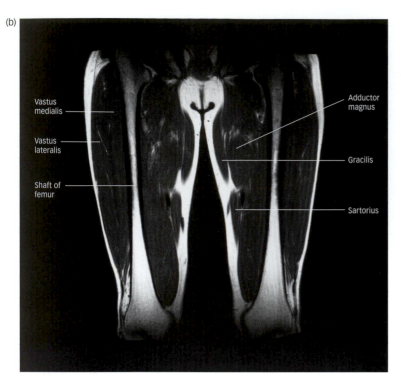

Fig. 13.10. *Continued*

trochanter and the linea aspera. Adductor longus arises from the front of the body of the pubis and is inserted by a broad aponeurosis on to the linea aspera. Adductor brevis takes origin from the inferior ramus and body of the pubis behind pectineus and is attached between the lesser trochanter and the linea aspera. Adductor magnus arises from the inferior ischio-pubic ramus and is attached along the linea aspera, the medial supracondylar line and by a strong tendon to the adductor tubercle of the medial femoral condyle. Its distal attachment is interrupted by the adductor hiatus through which the femoral vessels pass to reach the popliteal fossa, as the popliteal artery and vein.

The hamstrings

Semimembranosus arises by a flattened "membranous" tendon from the ischial tuberosity. It has a complex distal attachment to the medial tibial condyle and the medial surface of the tibia with tendinous expansions over the popliteus muscle to the lateral femoral condyle (the oblique popliteal ligament) and to the tibial collateral ligament (the posterior oblique ligament).

Semitendinosus takes origin from the ischial tuberosity. Inferiorly, its long tendon passes round the medial tibial condyle and over the medial collateral ligament to attach to the medial surface of the tibia posterior to the insertions of gracilis and sartorius.

Biceps femoris arises by a long head from the ischial tuberosity and a short head from the shaft of the femur. Its tendon inserts on to the head of the fibula.

The knee joint

The knee is a modified hinge joint and this synovial joint is the largest in the body. Although contained within a single joint cavity, the knee effectively comprises two condylar joints between the femoral and corresponding tibial condyles and a saddle joint between the patella and the femur. The tibiofemoral compartments are each divided by a fibrocartilaginous meniscus (Fig. 13.11). The medial meniscus is larger and more semicircular. It is broader and thicker posteriorly. The lateral is smaller, thicker and forms a nearly complete ring. The anterior and posterior horns of the menisci are attached to the intercondylar area. The posterior horn of the lateral meniscus is also commonly attached to the medial condyle of the femur by the meniscofemoral ligament. The transverse ligament joins the anterior ends of the menisci.

The fibrous capsule is attached around the margins of the articular surfaces.

The synovial membrane lines the fibrous capsule, but does not cover the surfaces of the menisci. It lines the suprapatellar bursa, which may be regarded as part of the knee joint and lies beneath quadriceps femoris, extending 7–8 cm above the upper border of the patella. Below the patella, the synovium is separated from the patellar tendon by the infrapatellar (Hoffa's) fat pad.

Posteriorly, the synovium is reflected anteriorly from the fibrous capsule to cover both cruciate ligaments on their anterior and lateral aspects. Several bursae surround the knee (Fig. 13.12).

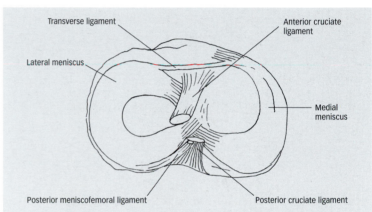

Fig. 13.11. **The menisci and ligaments of the knee and their attachments**

(a)

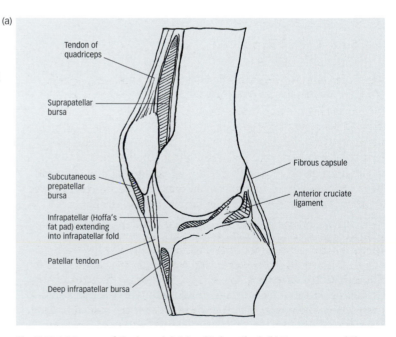

Fig. 13.12. **(a) Bursae of the knee joint (sagittal section); (b) Bursae around the knee; sagittal and axial MR arthrogram.**

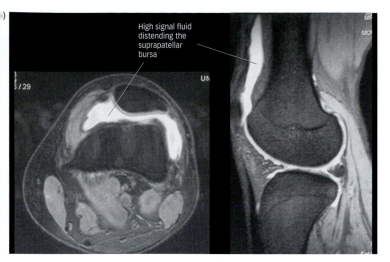

High signal fluid
distending the
suprapatellar
bursa

Fig. 13.12. *Continued*

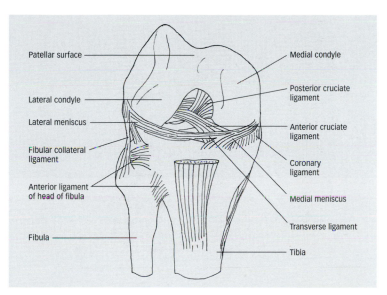

Fig. 13.13. **Ligaments of the knee Joints**.

The knee joint is strengthened by four main ligaments, (Figs. 13.13, 13.16). The medial (tibial) collateral ligament is attached to the medial epicondyle of the femur and to the medial tibial condyle. It is a flattened band, which blends posteriorly with the fibrous capsule, but anteriorly may be separated from it by a bursa. The posterolateral complex is made up of the popliteus tendon, biceps tendon, fibular collateral ligament, arcuate ligament, and popliteo-fibular ligament. The lateral (fibular) collateral ligament is a cord-like structure between the lateral epicondyle of the femur and the head of the fibula. Popliteus muscle arises from the posterior surface of the tibia and sweeps superolaterally behind the knee joint, where its tendon pierces the capsule and inserts in the groove on the lateral femoral condyle. Some of its fibers blend with the edge of the lateral meniscus. It also gives a slip to the tip of the fibula (popliteo-fibular ligament).

The cruciate ligaments (Figs. 13.13, 13.16), are intracapsular but extrasynovial. The anterior cruciate ligament (ACL) passes from the medial part of the anterior intercondylar area of the tibia upwards, backwards and laterally to insert into the posterior part of the medial

surface of the lateral femoral condyle. It prevents the femur moving backwards on the tibia. The posterior cruciate ligament (PCL) is attached to the posterior intercondylar area of the tibia and passes forwards, upwards, and medially to insert into the anterior part of the lateral surface of the medial femoral condyle. It is stronger and shorter than the ACL and limits posterior sliding of the tibia on the femur.

Movements

- *Flexion*: biceps, semitendinosus, semimembranosus. The extended knee is unlocked prior to flexion by popliteus, whose action is to rotate the femur laterally on the fixed tibia;
- *Extension*: quadriceps femoris;
- *Medial rotation of the flexed leg*: semimembranosus and semit-endinosus;
- *Lateral rotation of the flexed leg*: biceps femoris.

Imaging of the knee

Plain radiography (Fig. 13.14), is able to demonstrate the bony contours of the joint space. The normal tibio-femoral and patello-femoral joint space is 3 mm. The fat around the joint enables visualization of the patellar tendon, and allows an assessment of the presence or absence of a joint effusion. If a horizontal beam lateral radiograph is taken, a fat-fluid level (lipohaemarthrosis) in the suprapatellar bursa indicates a fracture within the joint. Occult fractures are usually of the tibial plateau. These may be demonstrated by coronal tomography or by thin slice axial CT with coronal reformatting.

If an abnormality of the patella is suspected, it should be imaged by the "skyline" view, a tangential view taken with the knee flexed. The intercondylar fossa of the lower femur may be imaged by the "tunnel" view, which is used to detect clinically suspected intra-articular loose bodies (Fig. 13.15).

MRI is much the most useful imaging technique (Fig. 13.16). It demonstrates the joint cavity, menisci, ligaments, and articular cartilage very well.

Dynamic scanning of the knee is also possible with modern scanners, which allow assessment of patellar tracking.

(a)

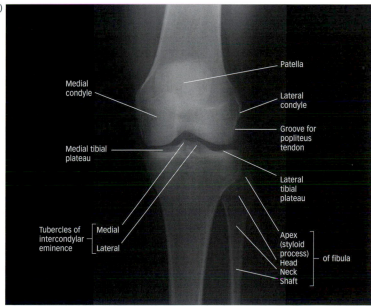

Fig. 13.14. **(a) AP, and (b) lateral radiographs of the knee.**

(b)

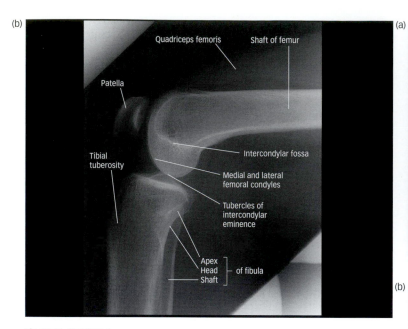

Fig. 13.14. *Continued*

(a)

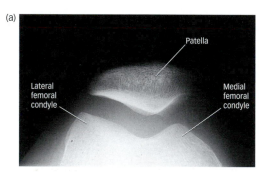

(b)

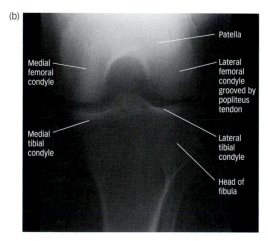

Fig. 13.15. **(a). A skyline view of the patella. Note how the lateral femoral condyle projects more anteriorly, tending to prevent lateral patellar dislocation; (b) intercondylar view of the knee.**

(a)

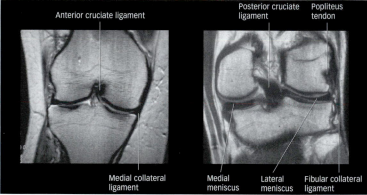

(b)

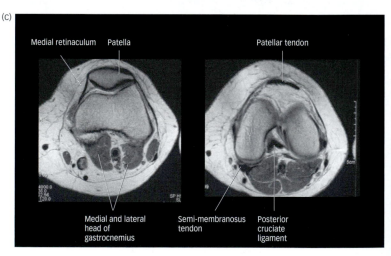

(c)

Fig. 13.16. **PD MRI of the knee (a) sagittal; (b) coronal; (c) axial.**

Ultrasound scanning may be used to assess the patellar tendon, the collateral ligaments and meniscal and popliteal cysts.

The lower leg

The tibia and fibula (Fig. 13.17)
These are joined by a tough fibrous interosseous membrane. They give rise to the attachments of many of the muscles of the lower leg.

Ossification is shown in Fig. 13.18.

The tibiofibular joints
The superior tibiofibular joint is a plane synovial joint between the head of the fibula and the articular surface under the lateral tibial condyle.

The inferior tibiofibular joint is a fibrous joint (syndesmosis) between the lower end of the fibula and the fibular notch of the tibia.

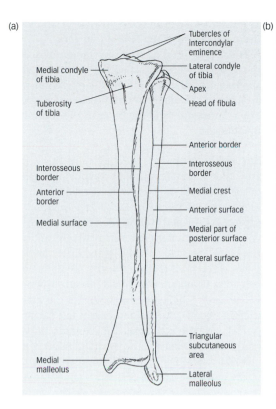

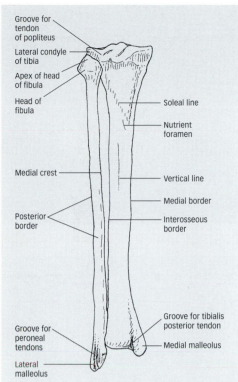

Fig. 13.17. **The tibia and fibula; (a) anterior, (b) posterior.**

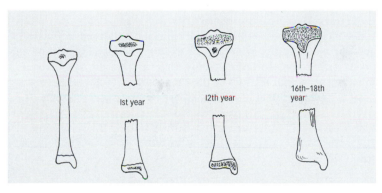

Fig. 13.18. **Ossification of the tibia and fibula. The distal and proximal epiphyses fuse with the shaft at 16–18 years.**

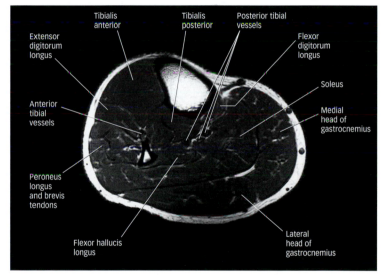

Fig. 13.19. **T1W axial MRI of the mid-calf.**

It is reinforced by the interosseous ligament of the joint and the anterior and posterior inferior tibiofibular ligaments. Movements at both joints are extremely limited.

The muscles of the lower leg (Figs. 13.19, 13.20)
Anterior compartment

Tibialis anterior takes origin from the upper part of the anterior surface of the tibia and adjacent interosseous membrane and forms a tendon which descends anterior to the ankle joint deep to the extensor retinaculum to attach to the medial cuneiform and the base of the first metatarsal.

Extensor hallucis longus (EHL) arises from the anterior surface of the fibula. Its tendon passes under the extensor retinaculum and inserts on to the dorsum of the base of the distal phalanx of the hallux.

Extensor digitorum longus arises above and lateral to EHL from the anterior surface of the fibula. Distally, it divides into four

tendons, which pass under the extensor retinaculum and insert via a dorsal expansion onto the dorsum of the middle and distal phalanges of the lateral four toes. Peroneus tertius arises from the anterior surface of the fibula and inserts into the shaft of the fifth metatarsal.

The lateral (peroneal) compartment

These muscles arise from the lateral surface of the fibula. Distally, the tendon of peroneus longus passes behind the lateral malleolus beneath the peroneal retinaculum, passes forwards lateral to the calcaneus and into a groove in the inferior surface of the cuboid

(a)

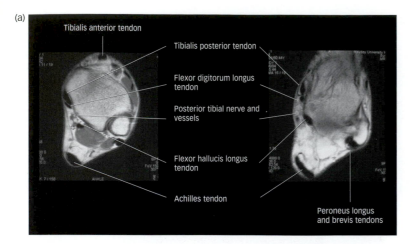

Tibialis anterior tendon

Tibialis posterior tendon

Flexor digitorum longus tendon

Posterior tibial nerve and vessels

Flexor hallucis longus tendon

Achilles tendon

Peroneus longus and brevis tendons

(b)

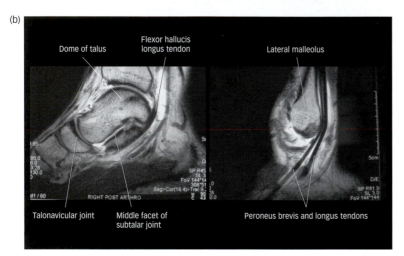

Dome of talus

Flexor hallucis longus tendon

Lateral malleolus

Talonavicular joint

Middle facet of subtalar joint

Peroneus brevis and longus tendons

Fig. 13.20. **PD MRI of the ankle. (a) axial; (b) sagittal.**

before inserting on the base of the first metatarsal and the adjacent medial cuneiform.

The tendon of peroneus brevis descends anteriorly to that of peroneus longus to insert on the base of the fifth metatarsal.

The posterior compartment.

Gastrocnemius, the most superficial of the muscles of the calf, arises by two heads from the posterior surfaces of the medial and lateral femoral condyles. A sesamoid bone, the fabella, is frequently found in the lateral head of gastrocnemius.

Soleus arises from the upper posterior surface of the fibula and from the posterior surface of the tibia. The tendons of gastrocnemius and soleus unite to form the Achilles' (or calcaneal) tendon, the thickest and strongest tendon in the body.

Flexor hallucis longus (FHL) takes origin from the posterior surface of the fibula. Its tendon descends behind the lower tibia and talus and under the sustentaculum tali, passing forward into the fibrous sheath of the hallux and attaches to the base of its distal phalanx.

Flexor digitorum longus (FDL) arises from the posterior aspect of the tibia. Its tendon descends behind the medial malleolus and then passes under the sustentaculum tali into the foot, crossing the tendon

of FHL (at the so-called Knot of Henry), and giving four slips to the distal phalanges of the lateral four toes.

Tibialis posterior arises from the interosseous membrane and the adjacent posterior aspects of the tibia and fibula. Its tendon shares a groove under the medial malleolus with that of FDL and attaches to the tuberosity of the navicular, giving slips to the other cuneiforms and the bases of the second, third, and fourth metatarsals.

The ankle joint

The ankle joint (Fig. 13.20), is a synovial hinge joint between the dome of the talus and the concavity formed by the medial and lateral malleoli and the inferior articular surface (plafond) of the tibia. The fibrous capsule is attached around the articular margins except anteriorly, where its attachment extends down the anterior surface of the neck of the talus. The synovial membrane lines the fibrous capsule.

The ankle joint is strengthened medially by the deltoid or medial collateral ligament, which has three components attached above to the medial malleolus and below to the tuberosity of the navicular (tibionavicular), the sustentaculum tali of the calcaneum (tibiocalcaneal), and the medial side of the talus and its medial tubercle (posterior tibiotalar). The lateral ligament complex is made up of the anterior talofibular ligament, joining the lateral malleolus to the neck of the talus, the calcaneofibular ligament, joining the lateral malleolus to the tubercle on the lateral side of the calcaneum (which is crossed by the tendons of peroneus longis and brevis), and the posterior talofibular ligament, which passes backwards from the lateral malleolus to the posterior process of the talus.

The movements of the joint are dorsiflexion, produced by tibialis anterior, extensor digitorum longus, extensor hallucis longus, and peroneus tertius, and plantarflexion produced in the main by gastrocnemius and soleus but assisted by the three other muscles of the posterior compartment of the leg.

The foot

The tarsus consists of seven bones arranged in three rows as demonstrated in Fig. 13.21.

The talus

This bone, which bears no muscle attachments, is made up of a body, neck, and head (Fig. 13.22).

The calcaneum

This, the largest of the tarsal bones, is irregularly cuboidal in shape with its long axis directed forwards upwards and slightly laterally (Fig. 13.23).

The navicular

The proximal surface articulates with the talus. The distal surface is divided into three facets for articulation with the three cuneiform bones. The lateral surface may have an articular surface for the cuboid. The medial surface bears a tuberosity, which is the principal insertion of the tibialis posterior tendon.

The cuneiform bones

These are bones lying between the navicular and the bases of the first three metatarsals. The medial cuneiform is the largest of the three

(a)

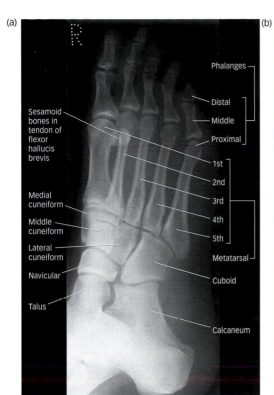

(b)

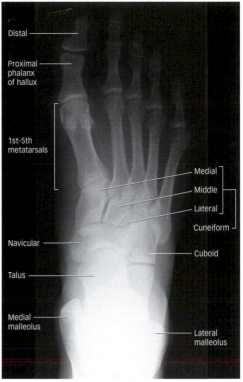

Phalanges
Distal
Middle
Proximal

Sesamoid bones in tendon of flexor hallucis brevis

1st
2nd
3rd
4th
5th

Metatarsal

Cuboid

Medial cuneiform

Middle cuneiform

Lateral cuneiform

Navicular

Talus

Calcaneum

Distal

Proximal phalanx of hallux

1st-5th metatarsals

Medial
Middle
Lateral
Cuneiform

Cuboid

Navicular

Talus

Medial malleolus

Lateral malleolus

Fig. 13.21. **(a) Oblique, and (b) dorsiplantar radiograph of the foot.**

(a)

(b)

(c)

(d)

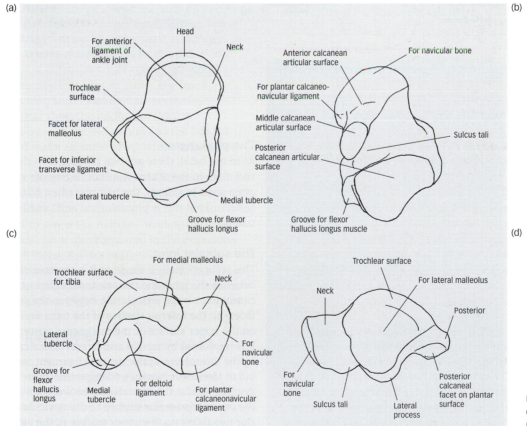

Head

Neck

For anterior ligament of ankle joint

Trochlear surface

Facet for lateral malleolus

Facet for inferior transverse ligament

Lateral tubercle

Medial tubercle

Groove for flexor hallucis longus

Anterior calcanean articular surface

For navicular bone

For plantar calcaneo-navicular ligament

Middle calcanean articular surface

Sulcus tali

Posterior calcanean articular surface

Groove for flexor hallucis longus muscle

For medial malleolus

Trochlear surface for tibia

Neck

Lateral tubercle

For navicular bone

Groove for flexor hallucis longus

Medial tubercle

For deltoid ligament

For plantar calcaneonavicular ligament

Trochlear surface

For lateral malleolus

Neck

Posterior

For navicular bone

Sulcus tali

Lateral process

Posterior calcaneal facet on plantar surface

Fig. 13.22. **The talus: (a) dorsal (superior), (b) plantar (inferior), (c) medial, (d) lateral.**

(a)

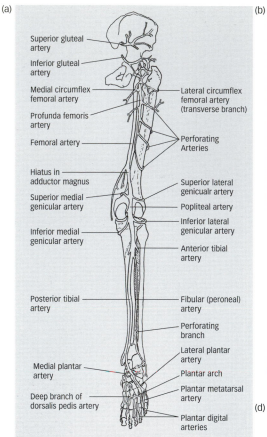

Superior gluteal artery
Inferior gluteal artery
Medial circumflex femoral artery
Profunda femoris artery
Femoral artery
Hiatus in adductor magnus
Superior medial genicular artery
Inferior medial genicular artery
Posterior tibial artery
Medial plantar artery
Deep branch of dorsalis pedis artery

Lateral circumflex femoral artery (transverse branch)
Perforating Arteries
Superior lateral genicular artery
Popliteal artery
Inferior lateral genicular artery
Anterior tibial artery
Fibular (peroneal) artery
Perforating branch
Lateral plantar artery
Plantar arch
Plantar metatarsal artery
Plantar digital arteries

(b)

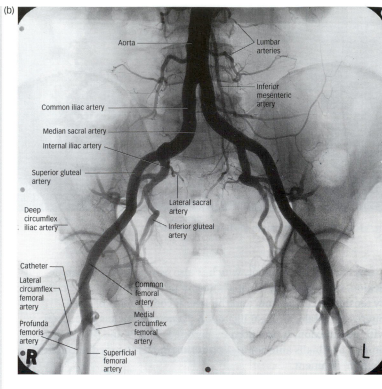

Aorta
Lumbar arteries
Inferior mesenteric artery
Common iliac artery
Median sacral artery
Internal iliac artery
Superior gluteal artery
Deep circumflex iliac artery
Lateral sacral artery
Inferior gluteal artery
Catheter
Lateral circumflex femoral artery
Profunda femoris artery
Common femoral artery
Medial circumflex femoral artery
Superficial femoral artery
R
L

(c)

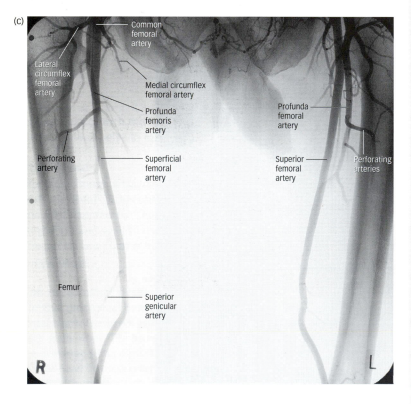

Common femoral artery
Lateral circumflex femoral artery
Medial circumflex femoral artery
Profunda femoris artery
Profunda femoral artery
Perforating artery
Superficial femoral artery
Superior femoral artery
Perforating arteries
Femur
Superior genicular artery
R
L

(d)

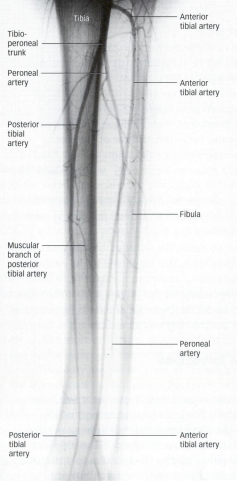

Tibia
Anterior tibial artery
Tibio-peroneal trunk
Peroneal artery
Anterior tibial artery
Posterior tibial artery
Fibula
Muscular branch of posterior tibial artery
Peroneal artery
Posterior tibial artery
Anterior tibial artery

Fig. 13.26. (a)–(d). **The lower limb arteries and arteriography.**

142

The external iliac artery becomes the common femoral artery at the level of the inguinal ligament. Just before this, it gives off the inferior epigastric artery and the deep circumflex iliac artery.

The common femoral artery gives off four superficial branches immediately below the inguinal ligament; the superficial epigastric artery, the superficial circumflex iliac artery, the superficial external pudendal artery, and the deep external pudendal artery. As it passes into the subsartorial canal, it gives off the profunda femoris artery and continues as the superficial femoral artery. The profunda femoris has six branches: the medial femoral circumflex artery which contributes to the supply of the hip joint, the lateral femoral circumflex artery, and four perforating arteries, which supply the muscles of the thigh. The supply of the femoral head is of importance because of its relevance to the management of femoral neck fractures.

As the superficial femoral artery passes through the adductor hiatus, it gives off a descending genicular branch and enters the popliteal fossa as the popliteal artery. This gives off seven branches to the knee joint and adjacent muscles as it descends behind the knee deep to the popliteal vein before dividing into the anterior and posterior tibial arteries. The posterior tibial artery descends between tibialis posterior and soleus muscles emerging on the medial side of the ankle joint posterior to the flexor digitorum longus tendon behind the medial malleolus deep to the flexor retinaculum where it is easily palpable. It divides within the plantar aspect of the foot into medial and lateral plantar arteries. The peroneal artey arises from the posterior tibial artery at the upper end of the fibula and descends towards the lateral aspect of the ankle. The anterior tibial artery pierces the interosseous membrane and passes forward into the upper part of the anterior compartment of the leg descending on the interosseous membrane crossing the anterior aspect of the ankle joint between the tendons of tibialis anterior and extensor hallucis longus. It continues into the foot as the dorsalis pedis artery.

Venous drainage

The deep veins of the leg correspond closely to the arterial supply with paired veins accompanying the major arterial branches. The superficial veins communicate with the deep veins via perforating veins which possess valves to promote drainage of superficial veins into the deep veins. The superficial veins also drain via the short (small) saphenous vein, which drains the lateral side of the dorsal venous arch and drains into the popliteal vein. The long (great) saphenous vein starts at the medial side of the foot, passes anterior to the medial malleolus, and passes up the medial side of the leg draining into the common femoral vein in the groin (Fig. 13.27).

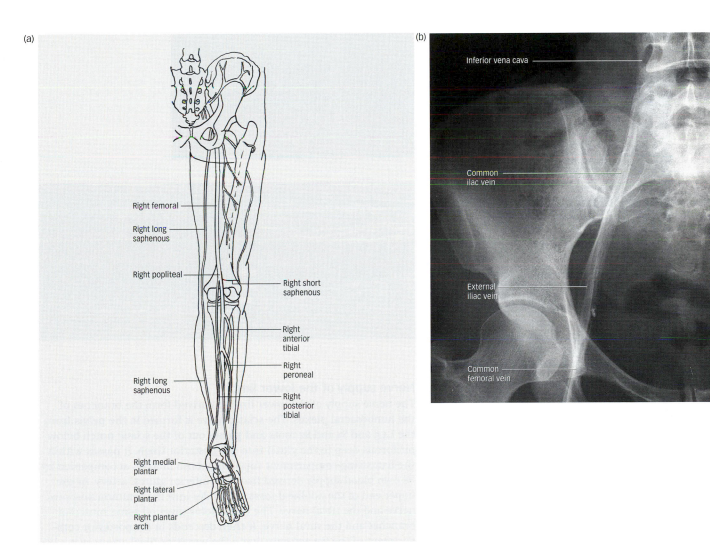

Fig. 13.27. (a)–(e) **The lower limb veins, diagram and venography. (f) Ultrasound scans of the femoral artery, B mode ultrasound and Doppler.**

143

provide a skeletal age by comparison with reference images. This technique is useful in congenital and metabolic conditions that alter skeletal maturation.

Knowledge of the appearances of epiphyseal ossification centers is useful in trauma, particularly around the elbow where an entrapped avulsed medial epicondyle may lie in the position of the trochlear ossification center.

Infantile bone marrow is hematopoietic and is of low signal intensity on MRI compared with the high signal fatty type seen in adulthood. During childhood, a gradual transformation to adult marrow occurs, beginning peripherally in the appendicular skeleton. The axial skeleton, including sternum spine and pelvis, retains hematopoietic marrow into adulthood. Longitudinal growth occurs at the physes or growth plates. These are highly vascular. Isotope bone scanning demonstrates markedly increased tracer uptake at these sites. When using these scans to look for bony metastases, osteomyelitis, or occult fractures, comparison with age-defined normal scans is essential (Fig. 15.9).

Index